Anna-Marie Lant

ELF-ASSESSMENT PICT  RY

Prosth

CW00547576

R.B. Winstanley

BDS, MDS, FDSRCS (Ed.)
Head of Department of Restorative Dentistry
School of Clinical Dentistry
University of Sheffield

M Mosby-Wolfe

London Baltimore Bogotá Boston Buenos Aires Caracas Carlsbad, CA Chicago Madrid Mexico City Milan Naples, FL New York
Philadelphia St. Louis Sydney Tokyo Toronto Wiesbaden

Copyright © 1994 Times Mirror International Publishers Limited
Published in 1994 by Mosby–Wolfe, an imprint of Times Mirror
International Publishers Limited
Printed by Grafos S.A. Arte sobre papel, Barcelona, Spain
ISBN 0 7234 1937 X

For full details of all Times Mirror International Publishers Limited titles,
please write to Times Mirror International Publishers Limited, Lynton
House, 7–12 Tavistock Square, London WC1H 9LB, England.

A CIP catalogue record for this book is available from the British Library.

Library of Congress Cataloging–in–Publication Data (applied for).

Preface

LIUBOV ANDREEVA 'Are you still a student?'
TROFIMOV   'I expect I shall be a student to the end of my days.'

The Cherry Orchard, I
Anton Chekhov

This series of questions and answers covers the general area of prosthodontics, including complete dentures and removable partial dentures, implants, diagnosis, occlusion, cosmetics, dental materials and dental technology.

The questions and accompanying illustrations have been submitted by experts in the subject areas and relate to commonly-encountered clinical situations.

Overlap with fixed prosthodontics is inevitable in such a text and serves to bring together the different specialisms that make up restorative dentistry.

This book will appeal to undergraduate and postgraduate students and those practitioners with an interest in prosthodontics.

Acknowledgements

The editor acknowledges, with grateful thanks, the time and effort generously given by Miss J.A. Newstead in preparation of the manuscript and the valuable assistance of the contributors in achieving deadlines.

List of contributors

I.C. Benington, BDS, FDSRCS (Eng),
FFDRCS (Irel), FDSRCPS (Glasg)
Department of Restorative Dentistry,
Queen's University, Belfast

P.V. Carrotte, BDS, LDSRCS (Eng)
Department of Restorative Dentistry,
University of Sheffield

R.G. Jagger, BDS, MScD, FDSRCS
(Ed) Department of Prosthetic
Dentistry, University of Wales
College of Medicine

R.B. Johns, PhD, LDSRCS (Eng)
Department of Restorative Dentistry,
University of Sheffield

A. Johnson, M Med Sci, LCGI, MCGI
Department of Restorative Dentistry,
University of Sheffield

D.J. Lamb, BDS, MDS, FDSRCS (Eng)
Department of Restorative Dentistry,
University of Sheffield

J.F. McCord, BDS, DDS, FDSRCS
(Ed), DRDRCS (Ed)
Department of Restorative Dentistry,
University of Manchester

S.E. Northeast, BDS, PhD, FDSRCS
(Ed)
Department of Restorative Dentistry,
University of Sheffield

R. van Noort, BSc, D Phil
Department of Restorative Dentistry,
University of Sheffield

G.E. White, M Med Sci, PhD
Department of Restorative Dentistry,
University of Sheffield

P.F. Wragg, BDS, FDSRCS (Ed),
DRDRCS (Ed)
Department of Restorative Dentistry,
Charles Clifford Dental Hospital,
Sheffield

1 A patient who has worn a complete upper denture for approximately 2 years complained of discomfort of the palate at the back of the denture, especially on swallowing.
(a) What is the lesion at the centre of the post-dam area?
(b) How was the lesion caused?
(c) What should be done about it?

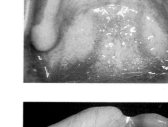

2 Careful inspection of this new complete upper denture will reveal a very small defect on the fitting surface of the left labial flange.
(a) What is it and how is it caused?
(b) What should be done about it?
(c) If undiscovered by the dentist, how will it affect the patient?

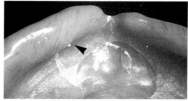

3 What are the uses of the surveyor?

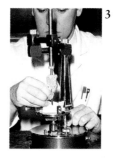

4 Calcium sulphate dihydrate has a spherulitic structure as shown on this scanning electron microscope view at a magnification of 2,500.
(a) Explain how it is that plaster expands on setting.
(b) How can the degree of expansion be controlled?
(c) In what dental applications is use made of the expansion characteristics of plaster?

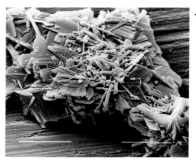

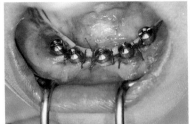

5 Why are healing abutments of the type illustrated sometimes used in place of conventional abutments at the second stage operation following the insertion of implant fixtures?

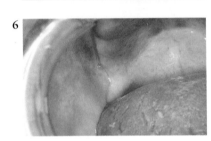

6 This slide shows the appearance of the mouth after removing the 10-year-old upper denture from an edentulous patient.
(a) What is the condition of the palate called and what organism may be associated with it?
(b) What systemic conditions may the condition be associated with?
(c) In the absence of any related systemic factors, how would you treat the condition?

7 The performance of a casting gold alloy, and therefore its clinical selection, is related to its mechanical and thermal properties. What type of alloy is indicated by the following performance data and what is the practical value of such data?

Melting range (°C)	Vickers hardness		Tensile strength (N/mm²)		0.2% Yield strength (N/mm²)		Elongation (%)	
	s	h	s	h	s	h	s	h
940–860	170	275	510	890	400	830	33	6

s = soft
h = hardened

8 The clinical appearance seen here was revealed following removal of a prosthesis.
(a) Name the design of prosthesis that has been removed.
(b) What has caused the soft-tissue lesions on the palatal mucosa?

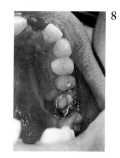

9 The patient illustrated has been edentulous for 10 years and, other than when attending important social events, has not worn his existing dentures. What problems do you foresee in providing such a patient with replacement complete dentures?

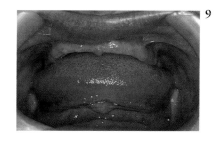

10 You are presented with a patient requiring complete maxillary and mandibular dentures. There is a Class 1 skeletal relationship. The maxillary ridge is level antero-posteriorly, with the mandibular ridge having a pronounced 'dip' in the premolar/first molar region, and a steep slope upwards in the second/third molar region as illustrated.
(a) How many posterior teeth would you use in the mandible and why?
(b) What teeth/ridge relationships would you use to ensure lower denture stability?
(c) How could you reduce the amount of pressure on the underlying tissue and bone from occlusal and masticatory forces exerted on the lower denture?

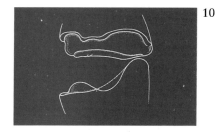

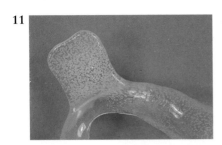

11 (a) What error can be seen in this heat-cured acrylic resin special tray, which typifies faults that can occur when processing acrylic resin?
(b) When flasking and processing acrylic resin dentures in two-part flasks, one problem always occurs. What is it, and how can it be corrected?

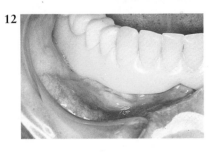

12 This patient presented with pain related to the lower denture for the past 3 months and an enlarged right submandibular lymph node.
(a) What is the cause of the pain and what is the nature of the lesion?
(b) Why does the patient have an enlarged lymph node?
(c) What should be the short- and long-term management of the situation?

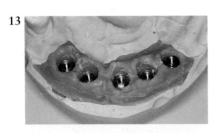

13 What are the benefits of using soft plastic or silicone material, as shown, around implant abutment analogues on working casts?

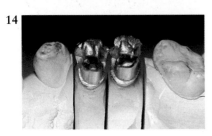

14 The gold crowns illustrated have been specially prepared in the laboratory.
(a) What features are shown and how are they prepared?
(b) What are the uses of crowns prepared in this manner?
(c) Describe the stages in planning and precautions that should be taken during tooth preparation when using such designs.

15 This 65-year-old lady presented with a history of persistent instability of her lower denture, the problem being most severe when eating. Five sets of complete dentures have been constructed in the last 10 years and all have proven unsatisfactory.
(a) Outline the possible causes of the lower denture instability.
(b) What examinations would you make to diagnose the causes of instability?
(c) How would you determine whether to modify or remake the complete dentures?

 15 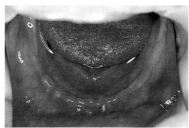 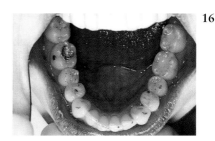 16

16 The colours shown on these teeth were produced after fitting and adjustment of the restorations.
(a) Describe how the different marks on the teeth are produced.
(b) What is the significance of the colours and distribution of the marks?

17 (a) What is the neutral zone?
(b) How can the neutral zone be recorded and incorporated into complete denture design?
(c) Describe how dentures constructed using a neutral-zone technique function.

A  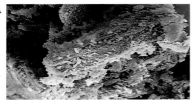 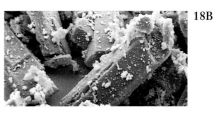 18B

18 Plaster (**18A**) and stone (**18B**) powder particles are illustrated under scanning electron microscopy.
(a) What are the production routes for plaster and stone?
(b) How do the resultant powders differ?
(c) What are the recommended powder/liquid ratios for plaster and stone?

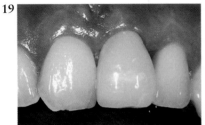

19 With the single tooth implant, what are the benefits of making a long-term temporary crown instead of completing the work immediately?

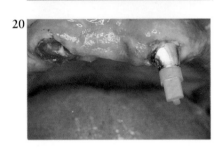

20 This patient attended with a loose partial overdenture, requesting improvement in the fit. The illustration shows one stage in the treatment of this case.
(a) What does the picture show?
(b) What is the function of the green coloured object on the tooth?
(c) What does the laboratory need to know before completing the repair?

21 What type of appliance is illustrated in **21A** and **21B**? Outline the possible uses of such a prosthesis and its design features.

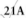

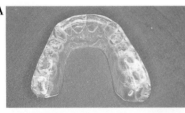

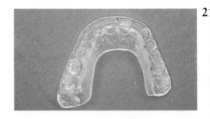

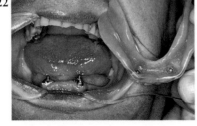

22 This lower overdenture is opposed by a natural dentition.
(a) How will this affect the overdenture?
(b) What precautions should be taken in designing the lower denture?
(c) What is the likely effect on the long-term management?

23 (a) What are the purposes of an impression tray?

(b) What are the advantages of a special (custom) tray over a stock tray?

(c) What factors determine the type of special impression tray you would request from the dental laboratory?

24 (a) Describe what is meant by the terms infra bulge and supra bulge when referring to clasps.

(b) Name three major connectors used in removable partial denture design.

(c) In removable partial denture design, what is meant by the term 'indirect retention'? Give an example.

25 What types of mouthguard are available for participants in contact sports?

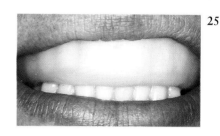

26 Given below are the constituents of acrylic resin denture base material. What is the function of each component?

Powder
(a) Polymethylmethacrylate beads.
(b) Benzoyl peroxide.
(c) Salts of cadmium or iron, or organic dyes.

Liquid
(d) Methylmethacrylate.
(e) Ethyleneglycoldimethacrylate.
(f) Hydroquinone (trace).
(g) NN¹-dimethyl-P-toluidine.

27 Comment on the acceptability of the acrylic resin partial dentures as illustrated in **27A** and **27B**.

A
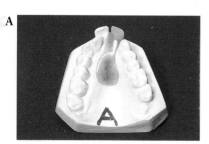

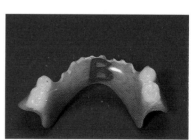
27B

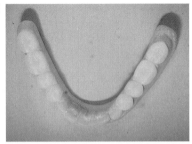

28 This complete lower denture belongs to a patient who complained of both generalised recurrent pain and looseness associated with the denture.
(a) What feature of the design contributes to the painful condition caused by the denture?
(b) What features probably contribute to the looseness of the denture?

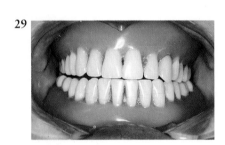

29 Examination of this patient wearing complete upper and lower dentures shows a premature contact on the left side with an occlusal space on the right in the retruded mandibular position.
(a) What difficulties might this occlusal error cause the patient?
(b) How might the defect have arisen?
(c) How may it be resolved?

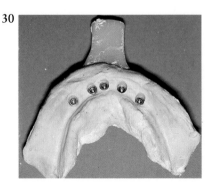

30 Why is a rigid impression material, such as the plaster illustrated, preferable to more elastic materials at the second impression stage of implant treatment?

31 This wrought overdenture retainer bar has fractured after only a short period of service. What could have contributed to this early failure and how may the fracture be repaired?

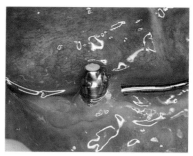

32 Adjustable articulators are intended to provide mechanical representations of jaws and temporomandibular joints and accurately duplicate their movements. In complete denture construction such articulators will help establish occlusal balance between the teeth. With these functions in mind why is it necessary for articulators to have incisal guidance tables when edentulous patients patently do not possess them?

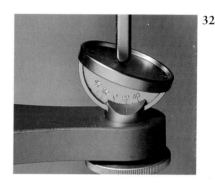

33 This flame-melted Type IV gold alloy casting shows surface pitting. How is this defect caused and which of the following remedial actions will prevent the fault occurring?
(a) Greater mould expansion.
(b) Thicker sprues/reservoirs.
(c) Increased casting force.
(d) Increased alloy casting temperature.

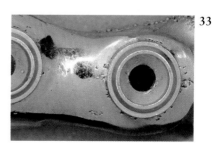

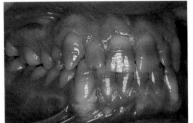

34 This patient, a 25-year-old male, complains that he is unhappy with the appearance of his teeth. What is the aetiology of this condition and how might it be managed?

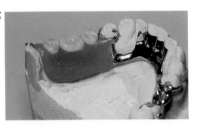

35 This lower unilateral distal extension partial denture has been waxed up ready for the try-in. What features of the design can be seen that will help to give a more stable finished result?

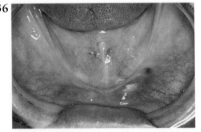

36 This patient has worn the same set of complete dentures successfully for 12 years, but for 3 days has had pain when eating.
(a) What part of the mouth is ulcerated?
(b) Why, with a history of this nature, is this part of the mouth more likely to be affected?
(c) What treatment is indicated before making new dentures?

37 This 50-year-old patient has retained only his lower anterior teeth, including the right first premolar and left first and second premolars. The lower central incisors are mobile and are painful to bite on. Radiographs show that the incisor and premolar teeth have little alveolar bone support. The canines, by virtue of their long roots, are well-supported. There is no caries. The patient requests restoration of appearance and function. What is the best form of treatment?

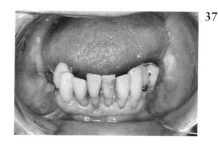

37

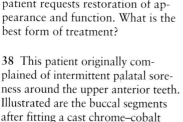

38 This patient originally complained of intermittent palatal soreness around the upper anterior teeth. Illustrated are the buccal segments after fitting a cast chrome–cobalt appliance (**38A, B**) and a view of the palatal surface (**38C**).

(a) Why might the patient be complaining of soreness behind the upper anterior teeth?
(b) Name the appliance that has been fitted.
(c) Describe the immediate effect of the appliance.
(d) What will be the outcome of wearing the appliance?
(e) Outline the long-term treatment options following appliance therapy.

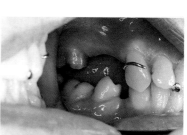

38A

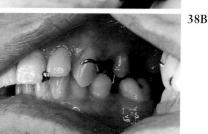

38B

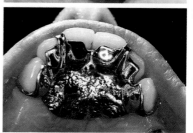

38C

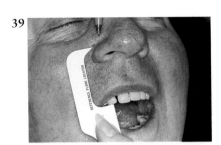

39 An important stage in recording a transfer using a maxillary face-bow is illustrated. What reference point is being established? How is this reference used during the remainder of the clinical procedures and what is its significance once casts are mounted on a semi-adjustable articulator?

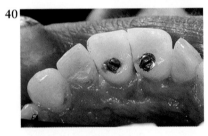

40 When a patient with a single tooth implant complains that the crown feels high even though it has been carefully adjusted to the occlusion, what might be the explanation?

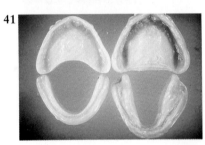

41 These two sets of complete upper and lower dentures were constructed for the same patient. The technique used for constructing the left set omitted one of the traditional stages in construction.
(a) Which stage in construction was omitted?
(b) What effects would this have on the dentures?
(c) How might the patient suffer as a result?

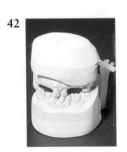

42 Study casts for a patient who requests a removable partial denture have been mounted on a simple articulator. What are the uses of these casts?

43 Should implants of the type illustrated be used to provide auxiliary support for natural teeth?

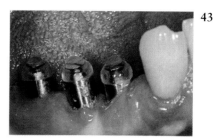

44 The durability of precision attachments relies upon careful case selection, design and application. The attachments shown here have been used to support an unusual anterior-saddle, lower removable partial denture, replacing the lower anterior and premolar teeth.
(a) What type of attachment is shown?
(b) Is the position of the attachments correct?
(c) How could the attachments fail in use?

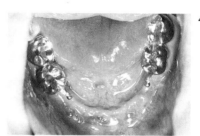

45 The occlusal records shown in **45A** and **45B** are sometimes taken in addition to a centric relation (CR) record. What relationships are being registered in each case and to what purpose are the records put when mounting casts on an adjustable articulator? Describe the limitations of such a technique in transferring the desired information.

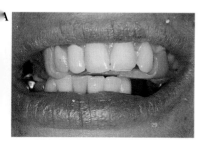

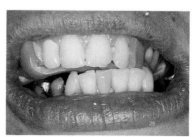

45B

46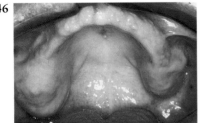

46 This upper edentulous ridge illustrates anatomical features that would cause difficulties in the construction of a satisfactory complete upper denture.
(a) What are these problematical anatomical features?
(b) What difficulties do they pose for the construction of a satisfactory denture?
(c) How may these difficulties be reduced?

47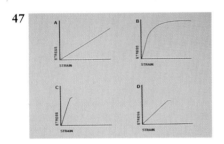

47 Using the mechanical property characteristics of rigid, strong, flexible, resilient, ductile, tough and brittle, which of these properties do each of the four illustrated stress–strain graphs indicate?

48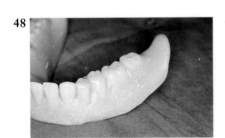

48 This denture was rejected by the clinician before it could be inserted into the patient's mouth.
(a) What defect does it demonstrate?
(b) What are the three most likely causes of the defect?
(c) What will the likely result be if the patient is allowed to wear the denture?

49 The patient depicted complains that the upper denture is loose. What are your observations and how do you explain the loose denture? What other factors may be important and what impression techniques might you use when treating such a case?

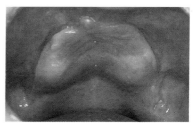

49

50 (a) Which of the clasp designs illustrated for distal extension prostheses will resist a vertical dislodging force most effectively?
(b) When designing distal extension partial dentures (Kennedy Classes 1 and 2), where would you place occlusal rests to best resist dislodging of the saddles in a vertical direction?
(c) What material would you use to construct a 'Roach arm' clasp?

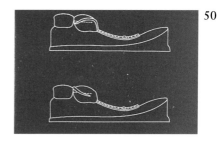

50

51 This edentulous mouth contains five osseo-integrated Branemark implants connected by a cast gold alloy framework.
(a) What is the purpose of such a framework?
(b) What are the likely consequences of fitting a prosthesis with an ill-fitting framework?

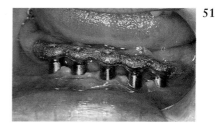

51

52

$$-\overset{\displaystyle CH_3}{\underset{\displaystyle CH_3}{Si}}-CH=CH_2 \quad + \quad H-\overset{\displaystyle |}{\underset{\displaystyle O}{Si}}-R$$

$$R-\overset{\displaystyle |}{\underset{\displaystyle O}{Si}}-H \quad + \quad CH_2=CH-\overset{\displaystyle CH_3}{\underset{\displaystyle CH_3}{Si}}-$$

$$-\overset{\displaystyle CH_3}{\underset{\displaystyle CH_3}{Si}}-CH=CH_2 \quad + \quad H-\overset{\displaystyle |}{\underset{\displaystyle |}{Si}}-R$$

+ platinum catalyst
⟶

$$-\overset{\displaystyle CH_3}{\underset{\displaystyle CH_3}{Si}}-CH_2-CH_2-\overset{\displaystyle |}{\underset{\displaystyle O}{Si}}-R$$

$$R-\overset{\displaystyle |}{\underset{\displaystyle O}{Si}}-CH_2-CH_2-\overset{\displaystyle CH_3}{\underset{\displaystyle CH_3}{Si}}-$$

$$-\overset{\displaystyle CH_3}{\underset{\displaystyle CH_3}{Si}}-CH_2-CH_2-\overset{\displaystyle |}{\underset{\displaystyle |}{Si}}-R$$

52 Illustrated is the setting process for an addition-cured silicone rubber impression material
(a) Addition-cured silicone impression materials come in a wide variety of viscosities. How is this range of viscosities achieved?
(b) What is the mechanism that converts the liquid polymer to a solid?
(c) Why must the impression be removed from the mouth with a short, sharp tug?

53
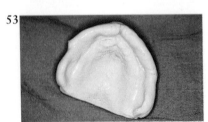

53 This impression has just been removed from the mouth.
(a) What problems might you expect when attempting to disinfect an alginate impression?
(b) What procedures may reasonably be used to disinfect an alginate impression?

54 One week after the insertion of this new cobalt-chromium based lower removable partial denture, the buccal cusp of an abutment tooth (which receives clasp arms and incorporates an occlusal rest) fractures. A crown is indicated and the patient cannot leave the denture. Outline how you can arrange for the replacement crown to 'fit' the denture.

54

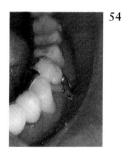

55 The provision of a complete upper denture opposing an almost intact lower natural dentition can pose many problems, particularly with regard to stability. Describe how you can 'customize' the denture to produce occlusal harmony for the patient.

55

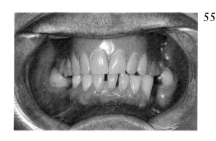

56 What is the amount of upper central incisor tooth exposure that is revealed below a relaxed upper lip in the natural dentition? What is the relevance of this to prosthetic dentistry?

57 The fitting surfaces of these metal-ceramic bridge retainers have been ground in the laboratory prior to delivery at the chairside.
(a) What could be the reasons for this metal removal?
(b) What is the likely consequence of this metal loss?

7A

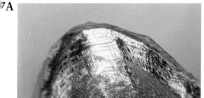

57B

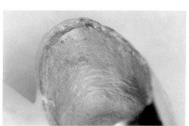

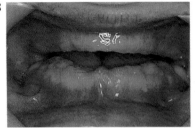

58 A patient requests provision of complete dentures following a dental clearance 9 months previously. With reference to the illustration, what problems do you foresee, and how might this affect your choice of materials for denture construction?

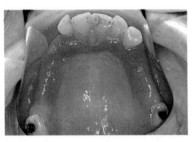

59 This patient complained of a burning sensation beneath her cobalt-chromium partial upper denture. Oral hygiene was good. Similar reactions were observed elsewhere when non-precious metal jewellery was worn next to her skin.
(a) What is the likely cause of the red area?
(b) What preliminary tests should be made to confirm this and what is the treatment?

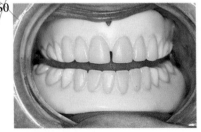

60 This patient complained of a gradual change in the colour of her dentures over a period of several years while using an immersion-type denture cleaner.
(a) What is the cause of the colour change?
(b) What change in denture hygiene would you advise for the future?

61 This patient complained of shortening of his teeth, problems with chewing due to loss of some posterior teeth and pain from both temporomandibular joints. The anterior teeth in their intercuspal position (ICP) is shown in **61A**. The right lateral view of the teeth in the same relationship is shown in **61B**. The retruded contact position (RCP) illustrates the large difference between RCP and ICP, **61C**. What investigations would you make before planning treatment? Outline a possible treatment plan for this case.

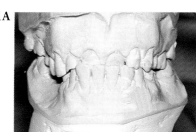
A

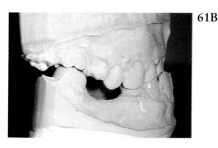
61B

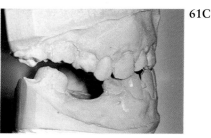
61C

62 What are the advantages and disadvantages of screw connection of a crown to an implant over cementation?

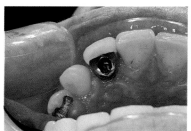
62

63

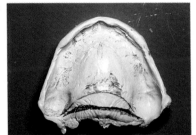

63 The illustration shows a rebase impression of a complete upper denture recorded in zinc oxide/eugenol impression paste, with the post dam delineated in indelible pencil.
(a) What was the patient's main complaint with the original denture?
(b) What design fault is evident from the photograph?
(c) What modifications are made to the denture before recording the impression?

64 How may cobalt–chromium castings be polished?

65

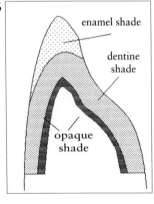

65 What type of working impression made for a removable cobalt–chromium-based upper removable partial denture is illustrated? What technique was used to make the impression?

66

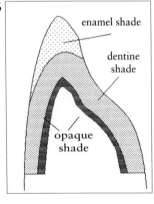

enamel shade

dentine shade

opaque shade

66 A porcelain jacket crown is constructed from opaque, dentine and enamel shades.
(a) How does the composition of the opaque porcelain differ from that of the enamel and dentine shades, and how does this affect its properties?
(b) Why are porcelain jacket crowns prone to fracture?

67 A metal–ceramic crown is up to three times stronger than a porcelain jacket crown.
(a) From where does the metal–ceramic crown derive its high strength?
(b) What is the most likely mode of failure with a metal–ceramic crown?

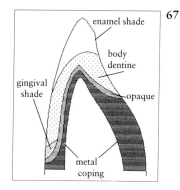

67

enamel shade
body dentine
gingival shade
opaque
metal coping

68 What are the advantages of overdentures over fixed prostheses in the implant-treated edentulous upper jaw?

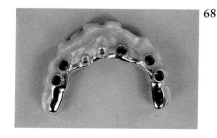

68

69 The complete dentures in the upper half of the illustration produced complaints, particularly of a painful and unstable lower denture. The newly constructed set (below) produced no such problems.
(a) What features of the troublesome lower denture account for the difficulties?
(b) How have these features been overcome in the design of the new lower denture?

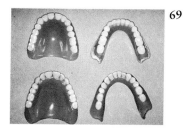

69

70

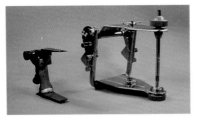

70 The majority of edentulous patients receive complete dentures made on simple hinge articulators (left). Knowing that most patients can manage dentures with cuspal interferences and that natural teeth are not occlusally balanced, why is it still desirable to use an articulator that simulates jaw movements more naturally (right)?

71

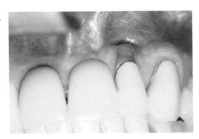

71 This 35-year-old patient presented complaining of the appearance of his front tooth which some months ago had been apicectomied. The tooth was an abutment for a three-unit cantilever bridge replacing a missing upper-left central incisor. A similar but satisfactory bridge was present on the right-hand side, replacing the missing upper right central incisor.
(a) What is likely to be seen on a periapical radiograph of the left lateral incisor and what is the prognosis for this tooth?
(b) List the possible treatment options to correct the problem.

72

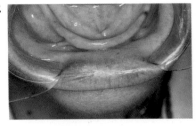

72 This patient complains of pain from her lower lip after eating. A linear zone of inflammation can be seen immediately behind the junction between the mucosa and the transitional epithelium of the lip. She has recently had new complete dentures made and asked for the lower incisors to be more prominent.
(a) What is the cause of the pain?
(b) How may it be corrected?

73 (a) What was the incisor relationship of this patient's natural teeth?
(b) Why are the incisors set in this way?
(c) Is a balanced occlusion achievable in this case?

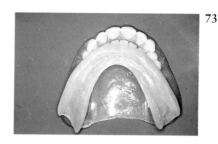

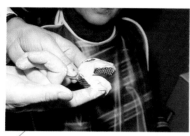

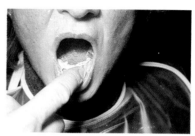

74B

74 What is being demonstrated here and why? (Please note that gloves should be worn routinely.)

75 A variety of metal alloys are used in the construction of restorations.
(a) What is an alloy?
(b) An alloy may consist of a number of different phases: what is a phase?
(c) In what forms may one metal be dissolved into another metal?

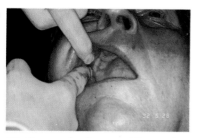

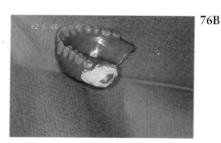

76B

76 One week after providing replacement complete dentures, this patient returned complaining of pain in the upper posterior segments on yawning or incising. This pain is not present when the upper denture is removed. What is the likely cause?

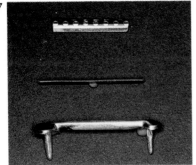

77 What type of precision attachment is demonstrated here? What factors determine the selection of this type of prosthesis?

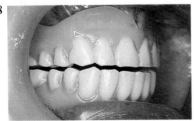

78 This patient complains of discomfort under the lower denture. What possible explanations are there and how might such a patient be treated?

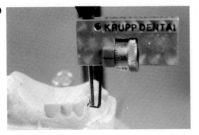

79 What is this device and how is it used? Give the main reasons for its use when surveying casts.

80 These dentures are occluding incorrectly at insertion when the patient is closing in the retruded contact position.
(a) What is the error and how has this unacceptable occlusion been produced?
(b) How may it best be corrected?

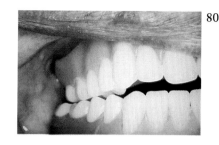

81 This illustration depicts the appearance of a 22-year-old female patient's teeth. What is the nature of this condition and how might it be treated?

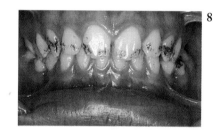

82 It is claimed that resin-bonded ceramics are less prone to fracture than porcelain jacket crowns.
(a) Why should this be so?
(b) How is the adhesive bond between the ceramic fitting surface and the resin luting cement achieved?

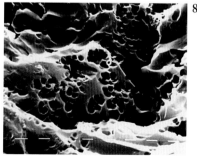

83 What are the possible causes of loosening of a gold screw in an implant-supported fixed bridge?

84 This edentulous patient complains of a loose lower denture and pain in the region of the right and left mental foramina. The pictures show the appearance with the upper denture only (**84A**), and the appearance with both dentures (**84B**). There has been moderate resorption of the alveolar ridges.
(a) What are the causes of the patient's symptoms?
(b) How would you rectify them?

84A **84B**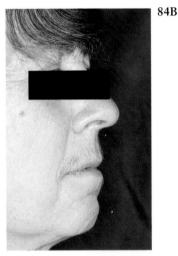

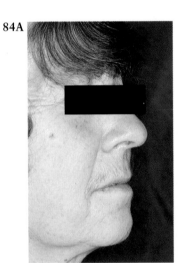

85 This appearance was observed 6 months after a course of dental treatment.
(a) What conditions are illustrated?
(b) Why has this occurred?
(c) What action would you take to remedy the problem?

86 This patient, who has been wearing the same set of complete dentures for 11 years, complains of a painful ulcer of the denture-bearing area in the lower left premolar region that has been present for 6 weeks. There is tender left submandibular lymph node enlargement. How would you manage the problem?

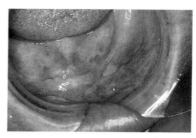

86

87 Why is it necessary to check the tightening of implant abutment screws at each prosthodontic stage of treatment, up to and including the final fitting of the prosthesis?

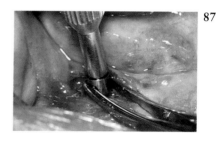

87

88 This patient requests a clearance and complete dentures. Consider how you might treat this case and what problems you might encounter.

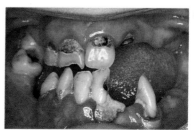

88

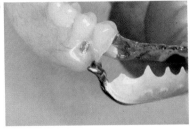

89 This lower removable partial denture demonstrates a particular retention system
(a) What is the system and on what principle is it based?
(b) When is it indicated in clinical dentistry?
(c) What options in design does it offer to fulfil particular clinical requirements?
(d) What are its disadvantages?

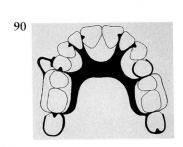

90 What faults are present in the schematic design of this toothborne upper cobalt–chromium partial denture intended for use in a correctly prepared mouth with adequately sound tooth support?

91 Upon smiling, an attractively natural dental appearance is obtained with artificial upper anterior teeth by duplicating which of the following lines?
(a) A line parallel to a line drawn through the pupils of the eyes.
(b) A line that is parallel to the lower lip.
(c) A line that is parallel to the upper lip.
(d) A line that is parallel to the inter-condylar axis.

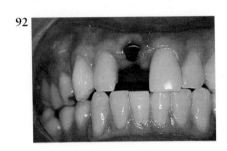

92 You have inserted an endosseous implant to restore this upper central incisor tooth. What restorative treatment options are available for temporary coverage during the healing (osseointegrating) phase?

93 This working impression in zinc oxide eugenol impression paste has the post-dam line marked in indelible pencil.
(a) Where should the post-dam line be positioned?
(b) How is the anatomical position transferred to the working cast?
(c) How does the clinician ensure a maximum peripheral seal along the posterior border?

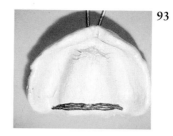

94 This is the upper edentulous ridge of an elderly patient.
(a) What condition is being demonstrated?
(b) What is the cause of this condition of the alveolar ridge?
(c) What problems does it present to the prosthodontist and how may they be minimised?

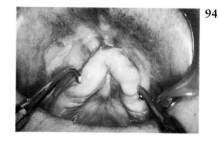

95 Four abutment teeth have been selected and prepared for this complete upper overdenture.
(a) What preparations have been carried out on each tooth?
(b) What factors would contribute to the retention of the denture?

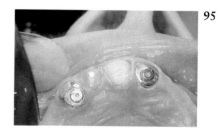

96 (a) What is the Bonwill triangle?
(b) How do the facebow and Bonwill triangle methods of mounting on the articulator differ, and which is preferable?

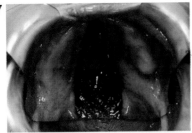

97 This 55-year-old edentulous patient has dentures that are now ill-fitting. His speech is poor and he queries whether or not you may be able to help. What problems do you foresee and what advice would you give this patient regarding treatment outcome?

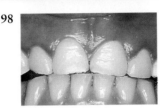

98 This illustration depicts the appearance of upper anterior crowns placed 24 months previously. The patient, in her early forties, seeks advice as to the nature of the problem and how it might be treated. What are your observations and what treatment will you offer?

99 Alginate:
(a) What is the setting process for an alginate impression material?
(b) What factors affect the dimensional stability of this impression material?
(c) What precautions must be taken when pouring a cast?

100 The typical compositions for conventional casting gold alloys are presented in the accompanying table.
(a) What is the purpose of the Ag, Cu, Pt, Pd and Zn alloying elements?
(b) What are the most appropriate applications for each of the four types of alloy?
(c) Why are hardening heat treatments of no use for Type I and Type II gold alloys?

Composition of conventional types of gold alloys

Type	Description	Au%	Ag%	Cu%	Pt%	Pd%	Zn%
I	soft	80–90	3–12	2–5	—	—	—
II	medium	75–78	12–15	7–10	0–1	1–4	0–1
III	hard	62–78	8–26	8–11	0–3	2–4	0–1
IV	extra hard	60–70	4–20	11–16	0–4	0–5	1–2

101 In the Nobelpharma[1] Cera One system, why is a gold alloy abutment screw used in place of a pure titanium screw?

[1] Nobelpharma AB, Nobel Industries, Göteborg, Sweden.

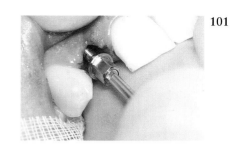

101

102 This patient complains that her right cheek is nipped by her new dentures
(a) What are the likely causes?
(b) How would you rectify them?

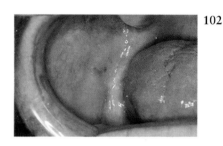

102

103 A patient complains of a tingling sensation beneath the upper complete denture that began 4 months ago when the denture was relined. The sensation has improved slightly with time. What is the cause of the complaint and how would you rectify it?

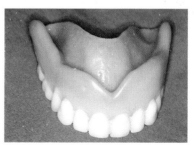

103

104 What is the reason for recommending a cure cycle for acrylic resin denture base material of 7 hours at 70°C plus 3 hours at 100°C?

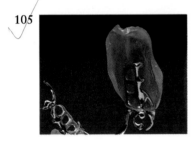

105 The acrylic saddle of this lower partial denture has been coated with impression wax using the Applegate technique.
(a) What is the purpose of this technique?
(b) What alternative techniques are available for dealing with the distal extension prosthesis?

106 What is a precentric record or check record? Describe a suitable method of making such a record.

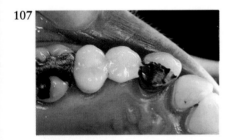

107 This illustration shows a 3-unit bridge replacing the missing upper right first premolar. A full crown metal ceramic retainer has been cemented on the upper right second premolar using conventional zinc phosphate cement. The three-quarter-metal retainer on the canine was cast in nickel–chrome alloy, electro-etched and resin-bonded to the tooth using the acid etch technique.
(a) How might the bridge fail?
(b) Criticise the design in relation to possible maintenance after failure.

108 The complete upper denture
illustrated is of a horseshoe design
to avoid the palatal lesion.
(a) Name the palatal lesion. What is
its nature?
(b) Does the palatal lesion's presence compromise the function of
the denture?
(c) If there is a problem with the
lesion's presence, how may it be
overcome?

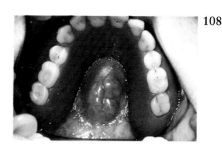

108

109 (a) What is the name and purpose of this apparatus?
(b) What may be the consequences
of not using this instrument?
(c) What other types of such instrument are there?

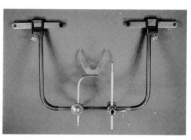

109

A

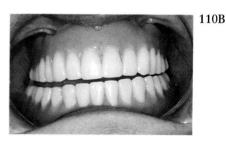

110B

110 This patient has complained of loose dentures since they were made 2
years ago, and has pain in the right temporomandibular joint region which
has gradually developed since fitting. The intercuspal position is shown in
110A and the retruded contact position is shown in **110B**. The occlusal face
height is correct.
(a) What is the likely cause of the patient's symptoms?
(b) What temporary measure would you take to correct the symptoms?

111

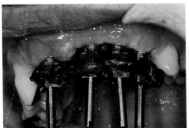

111 Why is it suggested that impression–transfer copings should be splinted together when a silicone impression is being taken for an implant-supported prosthesis?

112

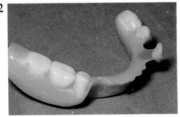

112 This partial denture has been made for a patient whose oral hygiene and periodontal condition is very poor. What is it called, and what might be its advantage?

113

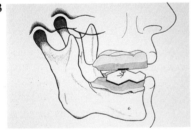

113 (a) What is the name given to the tracing being drawn and what is its purpose?
(b) What are the advantages of its use in the edentulous mouth during complete denture construction?

114 You have prescribed replacement complete dentures for a patient who has worn complete dentures successfully for 20 years. One month after insertion, the patient complains of a burning sensation in her/his mouth. Discuss what investigations you might make.

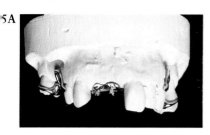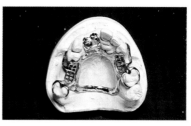

115 What design faults are present in these photographs of a chrome–cobalt base?

116 What are the likely causes of the palatal fracture of this denture?

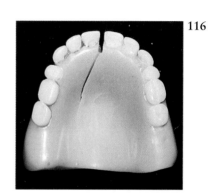

117 The picture illustrates a complete upper overdenture during construction.

(a) What exactly is the clinical stage being carried out with the permanent base *in situ*?

(b) What is the function and importance of the soft metal seen between the matrix and the patrix of the attachments?

(c) What anatomical feature indicates that the overdenture will require precision attachments?

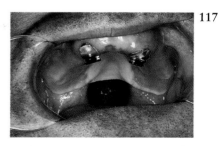

118

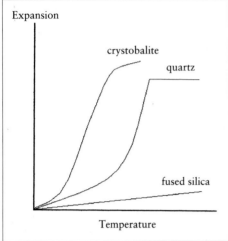

Expansion

crystobalite

quartz

fused silica

Temperature

A schematic representation of the effects of temperature on the expansion characteristics of three forms of silica.

118 (a) What are the two most commonly used investments and what alloys are they used with?
(b) The diagram shows three forms of silica. Why are crystobalite and quartz used in preference to fused silica?

119

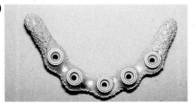

119 Describe the type of connector illustrated. What is its function and what problems are associated with its use?

120

120 On what basis is the length of the cantilever calculated in the edentulous lower jaw where 5 evenly spaced implant fixtures have been placed?

121 In this illustration, a corroded cobalt chromium full plate is seen with unaffected teeth and base. What has caused the condition?

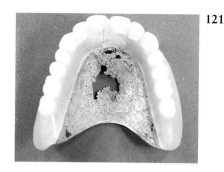

121

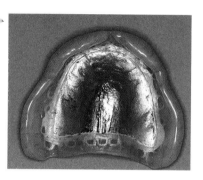

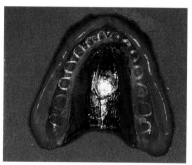

122B

122 Differing designs of complete upper dentures with cobalt–chromium-reinforced palates are shown in **122A** and **122B**. What are the advantages of **122A** over **122B** and why might metal reinforcement be indicated?

123 How is the casting shown retained on the tooth? Identify the important components of the design and describe their function. What alternative material could be used?

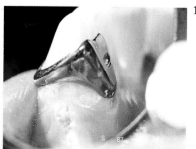

123

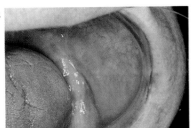
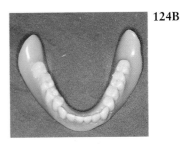

124 This patient has pain from her lower denture only when chewing, and a small ulcer is present in the left retromolar region (**124A**). After relieving the pain, the adjustment of the denture leaves a notch in the periphery in this region (**124B**). What was the cause of the pain in this area?

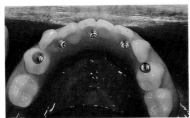

125 What precaution should be taken when sealing the access hole to the gold alloy screw in order to avoid damage to the head of the screw on removal of the implant retained prosthesis?

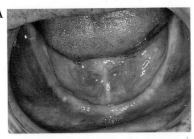
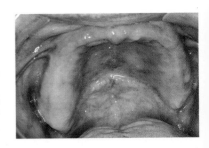

126 This edentulous patient, whose upper (**B**) and lower (**A**) denture-bearing areas are illustrated, complains of a burning sensation from the mouth, which is produced when the dentures are worn but which is relieved when they are removed.
(a) What is the likely cause of the burning sensation?
(b) How would you treat it?

127 This 5-unit resin-bonded bridge has been in place for 2 years. Debonding of the retainer from the canine abutment was noted at review.

(a) Why has the bridge failed at this position?

(b) Describe a more suitable design for this case.

(c) To what extent could you salvage the existing bridge?

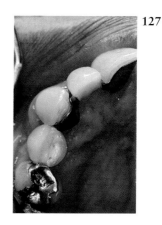

127

128 (a) What is seen in this radiograph?

(b) What related problems in prosthetic dentistry does this highlight?

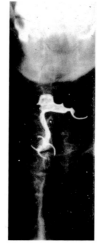

128

129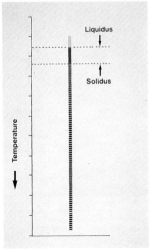

129 The graph shows an alloy heated to casting temperature immediately prior to casting. The yellow line indicates its superheated temperature range, the red line indicates the temperature range between the liquidus and solidus states and the black line indicates the solidus to room temperature cooling range. The alloy will contract as it cools through these temperature ranges. What mechanisms exist to compensate for these contractions so that an accurately fitting casting can be made?

130 What are copy dentures and how are they produced?

131 In metal-ceramic restorations the bond between the metal coping and the ceramic is of paramount importance to the longevity of the restoration.
(a) What 3 bonding mechanisms are involved in producing a bond between the metal and the ceramic?
(b) Why is the coefficient of expansion of the ceramic compared with that of the metal so important?

132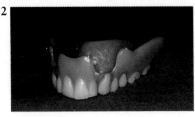

132 This upper complete overdenture has canine abutments.
(a) Why are the buccal flanges missing bilaterally?
(b) What adverse affects do the missing flanges have on the denture?
(c) How may problems caused by the missing flanges be compensated for?

133 The patient illustrated complains of a swelling in the lower anterior region that has been present for many years.
(a) What is the name of the condition?
(b) What is the cause of the condition?
(c) What treatment should the practitioner provide?

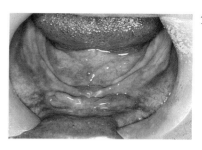

134 Describe the differences between using simple-hinge, fixed-condylar angle and adjustable-condylar angle articulators when constructing complete dentures.

135 What is the purpose of placing a reversed premolar behind the last lower molar when setting up on an articulator to an average condylar angle and mounting position for complete dentures?

136 What is the purpose of a stent in the upper anterior region during implant surgery?

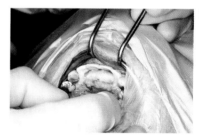

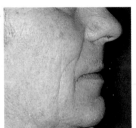
137A

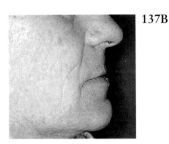
137B

137 This 71-year-old patient has worn the same complete dentures for 15 years and attends the surgery complaining that his appearance has deteriorated but that the dentures are otherwise satisfactory. The patient is shown at rest in **137A** and with his dentures in occlusion in **137B**. The difference between the occlusal face height and rest face height is about 12mm.
(a) What has occurred to account for the changes?
(b) How would you correct the complaint and what problems might arise?

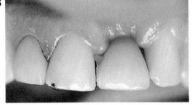
138

138 This minimal preparation bridge is being tried in before cementation. Describe the faults in the appearance of the pontic and outline how they could be improved. What could be done to improve the final aesthetic result prior to fitting the bridge?

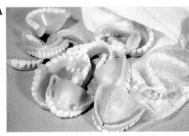
139A

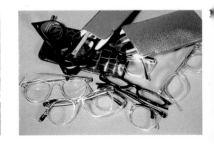

139 A patient presents complaining of inability to tolerate complete dentures that have recently been provided by another dental practitioner. A plastic bag containing several other sets of dentures (**A**) is produced by the patient who states that these have also been unsatisfactory. Another plastic bag, this time containing spectacles, is then produced (**B**) and the patient describes problems associated with wearing spectacles. What is the significance of this?

140 This 35-year-old lady complains that the upper left central incisor has discoloured following local trauma. Discuss the aetiology and consider how this might be treated.

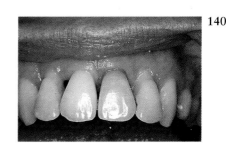

140

141 Illustrated is a hard palate defect resulting from a hemi-maxillectomy for the removal of a soft-palate salivary gland tumour that took place some 10 years ago. Discuss how you might construct a denture for such a patient.

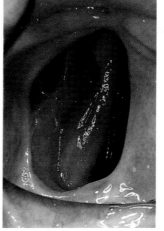

141

142 The single-implant-supported, upper central incisor may be thought of as a convenient introduction to implant dentistry. What factors may conspire to make this poor advice for the new implant team?

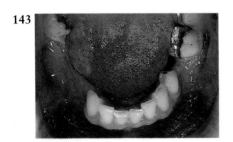

143 What factors do you see in this photograph that require attention prior to the recording of the definitive impression for a partial denture?

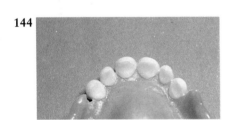

144 What type of prosthesis is demonstrated here? What design fault is incorporated? Discuss how you might effect a reline of this prosthesis.

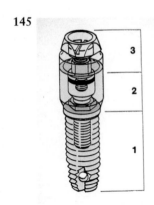

145 Shown are the constituent parts of a typical titanium dental implant.
(a) What are the functions of parts 1, 2 and 3?
(b) What is the function of the external implant threads?
(c) Why is it necessary to have a gold alloy cylinder rather than preserve an all-titanium external construction?

146 Investment moulds must expand on furnace heating by an amount sufficient to compensate for the contraction of cast molten metal on cooling. The investment shown in the graph has an expansion plateau between 450°C and 700°C, so accurate castings may be made anywhere within this temperature range. What other mould temperature control is necessary to ensure accurate castings?

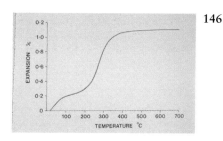

147 If, on seeing the patient after second-stage implant surgery, it is apparent that the abutments are at an angle that will require access cavities on the labial aspect of the teeth, what methods are available to deal with the problem?

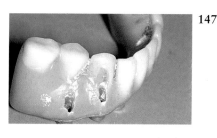

148 Illustrated is a common denture situation. What problems are often associated with it?

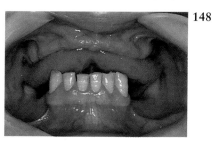

149 Dies for cast crowns are sometimes provided with a coating of paint.
(a) What is the purpose of such coatings and what should the extent of their coverage and thickness be?
(b) What faults may be indicated when the coating and die have been damaged as shown?

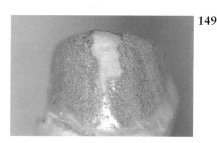

150 The quality of the masticatory function of a complete denture depends on its retention and stability.
(a) Define retention and stability.
(b) Explain what factors govern the retention of a denture.

151

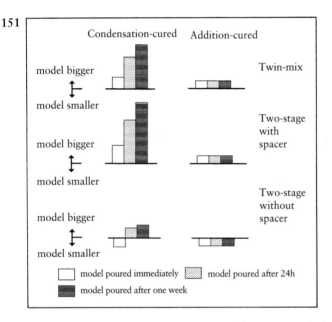

151 The diagram shows the effect of 2 different types of silicone impression material and 3 impression-taking techniques on the size of a cast poured. Explain how these dimensional differences arise and state which technique may be most appropriate for which type of impression material.

152

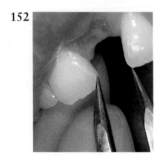

152 A patient requests that a missing upper central incisor be replaced with an implant. The space between the adjacent crowns is 6mm. What other information is required?

153 This patient complains of a loose upper complete denture.
(a) Why is the denture loose?
(b) What treatment is required before satisfactory dentures can be made?

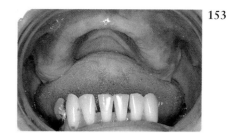

154 This edentulous patient has been a denture-wearer for 20 years and now complains of discomfort at the corners of the mouth.
(a) Name the painful bilateral condition.
(b) Is the bilateral condition associated with any intraoral condition, and, if so, what is it and how is it caused?
(c) How is the patient with this condition managed?

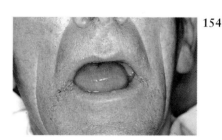

155 What is illustrated here and how can it be avoided?

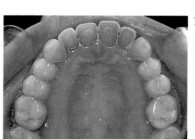

156 These are the anterior teeth of a 25-year-old female. She complains that these teeth are deteriorating and becoming increasingly sensitive. What is the possible cause of this condition and how might it be treated?

157 What is a castable glass-ceramic?

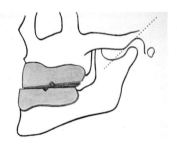

158 A protrusive jaw movement with occlusal rims in contact produces a separation posteriorly as illustrated.
(a) What causes this separation and what clinical use may be made of this effect?
(b) If complete dentures separated in the same way this would remove occlusal balance of the teeth. How may this tooth separation be avoided when setting the posterior teeth in complete dentures?

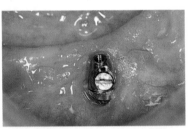

159 When placing an angled abutment, how may its correct position be maintained while tightening the abutment screw?

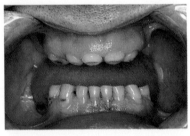
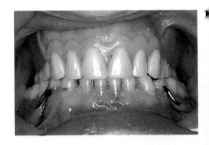

160 This patient has only upper and lower anterior teeth remaining and suffered severe upper anterior tooth wear over many years (**A**). He has now been provided with a complete upper overdenture and a partial lower denture (**B**).
(a) What type of abutment preparations were undertaken and why?
(b) Are precision attachments necessary to retain the overdenture?
(c) Why was a full labial flange contraindicated in this case?

161 The patient depicted here complains that his upper anterior teeth have worn away. Describe in principle how you might handle such a case.

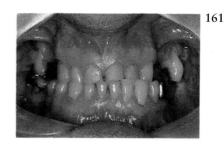

161

162 What technique is depicted here? What is its purpose?

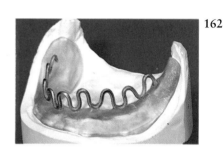

162

163 When finished complete dentures are presented on the articulator they are found to have an increased occlusal vertical dimension as revealed by a gap between the tip of the incisal guidance pin and its table. What circumstances could have led to this error?

164 Pins inserted into the abutment replicas in this master cast indicate the angulations of the implants installed in the patient's mouth. What are the advantages and disadvantages of such inclinations for the construction of the prosthesis that then follows?

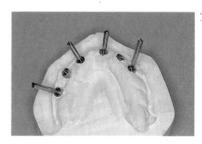

164

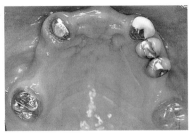

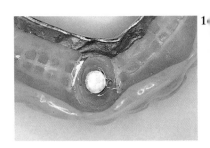

165 The cast restorations on the teeth shown in **165A** have been designed to support a removable partial denture (**165B**). What method has been used to retain the prosthesis over the upper right canine root?

166 What are the functions of a partial denture?

167 Describe Kennedy's classification of partial dentures.

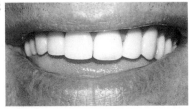

168 List the factors associated with this upper denture that compromise the appearance of the patient.

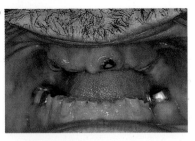

169 Why have these teeth been reduced in height? Discuss the advantages and disadvantages of this treatment option.

170 It has been confidently proposed that dental implants will form an increasingly widespread alternative to conventional single tooth restorations and complete and partial prostheses of all kinds. Why is it hoped that this forecast is incorrect?

171 This upper acrylic resin partial denture may be criticised in a number of ways. Which criticism do you consider to be the most important?

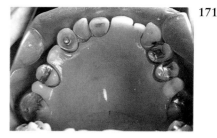

171

172 (a) Why has this complete denture been designed with a metallic base?
(b) What is the material of the metallic base?
(c) What other metallic base is occasionally used for constructing a complete upper denture and why?
(d)What is the difficult long-term problem in servicing this type of denture?

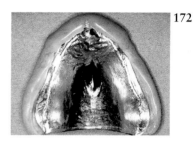

172

173 This patient has a partial upper overdenture.
(a) What is the probable reason for the upper anterior alveolar defect?
(b) Why have precision attachments been chosen for the abutments?
(c) Why is an overdenture indicated in this case?

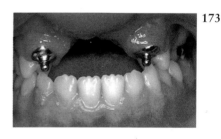

173

174 This patient was provided with new dentures 3 months previously but complains that the upper denture becomes loose, with loss of 'suction' when he bites. The ridges are well formed, denture extension is correct and the dentures are individually retentive and stable.
(a) What is the probable cause of the problem?
(b) How would you correct it?

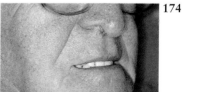

174

175 (a) Describe the two major causes of porosity in acrylic resin dentures.
(b) How may these problems be avoided?

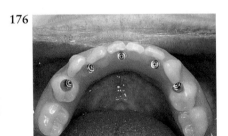

176 Implant-supported prostheses that are fixed in place in the mouth are connected to their supporting implants by means of small screws. Knowing that these screws can break in function, how should they be tightened to ensure a long service life?

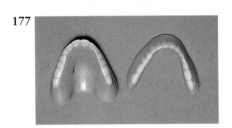

177 An elderly edentulous patient attends your surgery. She has worn her present dentures for 30 years and the occlusal surfaces have worn considerably. What difficulties might you encounter in recording the registration and how would you overcome them?

178 What is meant by the term undercut in relation to partial denture design?

179 Name the following dental materials:
(a) $CaSO_4 \, \frac{1}{2}H_2O$ $(CaSO_4)_2 \, H_2O$

(b)

	Kaolin %	Silica %	Feldspar %	Glass %
(i)	4	15	80	0
(ii)	0	25	60	15

(c)

	Au %	Ag %	Cu %	Pt/Pd %	Zn %
(i)	85	11	3	—	1
(ii)	75	12	10	2	1
(iii)	70	14	10	5	1
(iv)	65	13	15	6	1

(d) (i) Rosin, yellow beeswax, gum dammer.
(ii) Paraffin wax, beeswax.
(iii) Paraffin wax, carnuba, candililla, beeswax.
(e) Sodium or potassium salt of alginic acid, $CaSO_4.2H_2O$, Na_3PO_4, diatomaceous earth, reaction indicator.

180 (a) What is the likely prognosis of the lower denture illustrated? (b) What alternative measures should have been taken in this case?

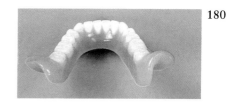

180

181 What factors would influence your choice of treatment options for a missing permanent maxillary central incisor?

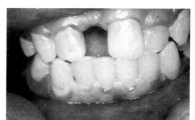

181

182 This mandibular impression was made in a 2-part impression tray designed to lock together in the mouth and uses 2 different types of impression material. It is primarily designed for taking impressions of Kennedy Class 1 and Class 2 mouth conditions.
(a) Why would it be advantageous to use this type of impression tray?
(b) What other commonly used method is available to achieve the same results as the 2-tray system?

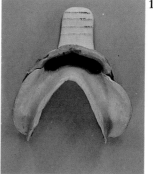

182

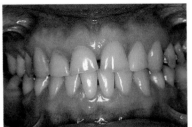

183 This 36-year-old female complains that her upper anterior teeth are beginning to shorten. What is the possible cause and how should it be managed?

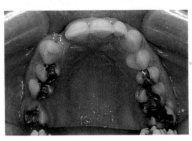

184 What are the alternative types of fixed replacement restorations for the missing right lateral incisor tooth? What problems may occur?

185 On occasions a patient may require a denture soft liner to overcome problems of persistent pain and discomfort with a complete denture.
(a) How does a soft liner help to improve the situation?
(b) What are the 2 major types of soft liner?
(c) Why is the lifetime of soft liners limited?

186 Describe the surveyor and the tools used with it.

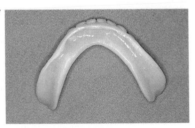

187 A patient complains that her lower complete denture (illustrated) is loose when eating and talking, and when she opens her mouth. There are no functional over-extensions of the periphery and both dentures are well retained. There are no obvious occlusal faults. What is the likely cause of the patient's problem?

188 This patient has been treated by means of a complete overdenture. What are the advantages and disadvantages of this form of therapy?

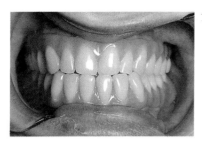

189 Owing to their brittle nature, ceramics are prone to fracture. This has led to the development of high-strength ceramics such as the ones illustrated in the table.
(a) What factors influence the strength of ceramics?
(b) Besides the introduction of a crystalline phase, what other mechanisms might be employed to improve the strength of ceramics?

Table of strength values for industrial and dental ceramics

Type of ceramic	Flexural strength (MPa)
Industrial	
Hot-pressed silicon nitride	800–900
Hot-pressed silicon carbide	400–750
Partially stabilized zirconia	640
Alumina 98% pure	420–520
Dental	
Leucite reinforced ceramic	60–130
Castable glass ceramic	120–140
Aluminous core porcelain	125–150

190 (a) Why do we construct special (custom) impression trays with differing thicknesses of spacer?
(b) What materials are available for the construction of special trays and what are their relative merits?
(c) What type of retention is required to retain alginate impression material securely within the tray?

191 (a) What fitting surface defects can be seen inside this metal-ceramic crown presented to the dentist by the laboratory?
(b) What are the clinical consequences of such defects?

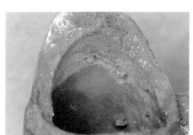

192

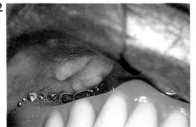

192 What is the swelling associated with the periphery of this denture? What is the cause and what treatment should be undertaken?

193 Describe why a cast should be surveyed during the design of a partial denture.

194

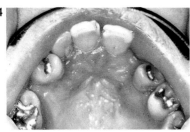

194 What is the cause of the diffuse redness seen in the palate illustrated?

195

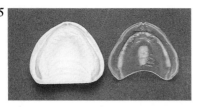

195 What is the purpose of this appliance? Discuss how you would manage such a case.

196

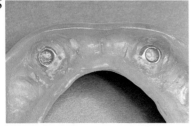

196 This overdenture is retained by precision attachments on the upper canine abutments.
(a) When relining the denture with a clinical reline material, what precautions need to be taken?
(b) If the overdenture is not relined to keep pace with alveolar resorption, what problems may occur?

197 What do you see of note in this radiograph? What has happened and why? What disadvantages may there be to such treatment?

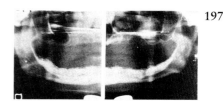

198 What instructions would you give your patient in how to care for this denture?

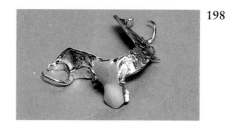

199 An elderly patient who wears complete upper and lower dentures, complains of pain in the lower jaw. Discuss possible causes of this pain.

200 (a) Give two examples of when it could be advantageous to tilt the cast to alter the path of insertion during the design of a partial denture.
(b) In partial denture designing, what are wanted and unwanted undercuts and how would you eliminate unwanted undercuts?
(c) How can a chosen path of insertion for a partial denture be transferred accurately and simply by the dentist to the technician?

201 What is the nature of this denture lining? How is it prepared and when is it not indicated?

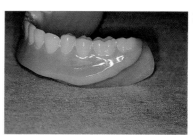

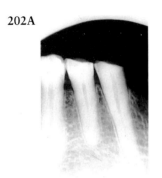
202A

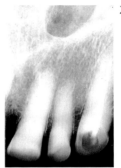
202B

202 These radiographs were taken of a patient referred for a clearance and provision of complete dentures. Why might this treatment plan cause problems if it is followed? What clinical condition might be present to account for the radiographic appearances?

203A
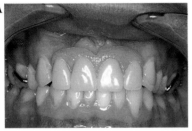
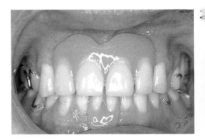

203 Illustrated are two examples of partial denture saddles with differing degrees of flange extension into the sulci. What factors have to be taken into account when deciding the depth of flange?

204
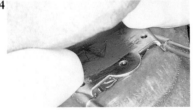

204 This patient has presented some difficulty at the registration stage for complete dentures in closing in the retruded contact position (RCP). What technique is being used here to enable the registration to be recorded satisfactorily? What other advantages does this technique offer?

205 The facebow illustrated will give the same information as that previously discussed in **109**. What additional information may be obtained compared with a maxillary facebow?

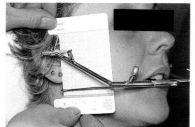

205

206 Rest seats for tooth-supported removable partial dentures are often not prepared when there is sufficient room from any opposing teeth in closure in the intercuspal position (ICP). Why should rest seats always be prepared?

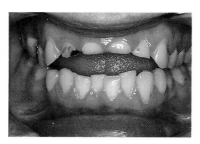
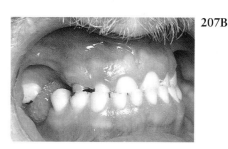

207B

207 Both patients illustrated exhibit marked tooth wear (tooth surface loss). The patient in **207A** complains of sensitivity of the affected teeth to hot and cold stimuli. The patient in **207B** does not complain of any sensitivity. Apart from individual variations in pain thresholds, why should this variation exist?

208 This patient has a large number of upper anterior teeth missing in an otherwise complete dentition. What are the possible restorative solutions for replacing the missing teeth?

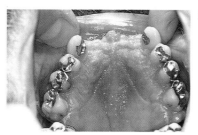

208

209 With reference to **208**, what advantages may a removable partial denture have over fixed bridgework?

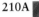

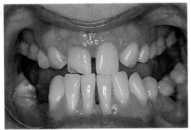
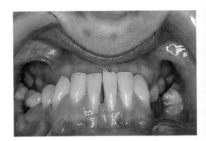

210A, B What is the significance of the two views of this patient closing together?

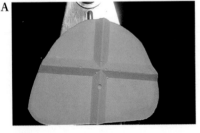

211 What is the most likely reason for the appearance of the incisal edges of the anterior teeth in this patient?

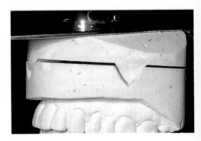

212 What technique is illustrated in **212A** and **212B**, and what may it be used for?

213 What problems do you foresee in replacing the missing upper anterior teeth in this patient?

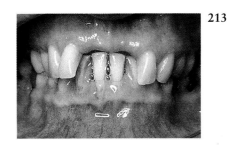

214 This appearance is not uncommon with a patient wearing a complete upper denture and lower bilateral free end saddle lower removable partial denture. What has occurred?

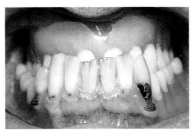

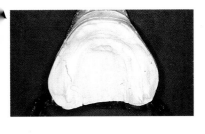

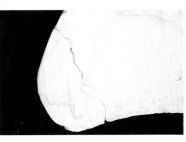

215 What is noticeable about this mounted cast for a complete denture and what will be the consequences if the defect is not remedied?

ANSWERS

1 (a)A small denture-induced ulcer with an associated nodule of hyperplastic tissue that has developed over a period of months.
(b)As a result of the posterior border of the complete upper denture being incorrectly designed – either the posterior border of the denture was over-extended beyond the vibrating line or the post-dam ridge on the fitting surface of the denture had a sharp posterior edge.
(c)The exact cause of the lesion should be ascertained and if the denture is over-extended it should be reduced carefully to eliminate the source of trauma. If the retention has been jeopardised by this alteration it may be necessary to replace the post-dam ridge using a clinical reline resin.

If, on the other hand, the lesion has been caused by the posterior border being too sharp, then it should be sufficient simply to smooth it carefully and then polish it.

The patient should be reassured regarding the benign nature of the lesion and reviewed in three weeks to confirm resolution of the ulcer. Occasionally the hyperplastic tissue may have to be removed if it continues to be traumatised by the denture.

2 (a) It is a small pimple of acrylic resin caused by a porous defect in the working cast. Small bubbles of air are easily trapped when pouring the working casts but this may be reduced to a minimum by using a vibrator or, better still, a vacuum machine.
(b) The technician should always scrutinise all surfaces of dentures carefully so that irregularities or sharp edges may be corrected before dispatching to the clinic. If undiscovered by the technician, it is the ultimate responsibility of the clinician to ensure that any surface defects on the prosthesis are modified appropriately before insertion in the mouth.
(c) This type of acrylic pimple is very sharp and will cause great discomfort to the patient in the early stages of wearing dentures, thereby creating the greatest psychological disadvantage. If the patient continues to wear the denture, which is unusual, a painful ulcer will develop.

3 The surveyor or paralleling device is used during both the diagnostic and construction stages of removable partial denture treatment:
(i) Soft tissue and tooth undercuts can be identified and marked.
(ii) The path of insertion can be decided and this may be marked with the surveyor on the casts.
(iii) The degree of undercut the direct retainers are to engage may be marked on the cast.
(iv) Blocking out unwanted undercuts in wax or plaster parallel to the path of insertion can be carried out.

See also **79, 186, 193** and **200**.

4 (a)On setting, the calcium sulphate dihydrate crystals that form are spherulitic in appearance, not unlike snowflakes. These crystals impinge on one another as they grow and try to push each other apart. The result of this action is that there is an apparent expansion on setting. The material in fact shrinks, in the sense that its molar volume is less, as shown below:

$$(CaSO_4)_2.H_2O + 3H_2O \rightarrow 2CaSO_4.2H_2O$$

Molecular weight	290	54	344
Density	2.75	1.0	2.32
Molar volume	105	54	148

Change in molar volume = $\dfrac{(148 - 159)}{159}$ = -7.1%

However, there are large empty spaces between the crystals. Thus the material is highly porous and this accounts for the apparent expansion.
(b)There are various additives in gypsum products to control the degree of expansion. The additives are:
● Sodium chloride. This additive provides additional sites for nucleation of the crystals. The crystals are more spherical and smaller and so do not push each other apart as much as larger crystals do, thus reducing the apparent expansion.
● Potassium suphate. Potassium sulphate (K_2SO_4) reacts with the water and hemihydrate to produce 'syngenite' ($K_2(CaSO_4)_2.H_2O$). This phase crystallizes very rapidly, to produce more crystals, and this again has the effect of reducing the overall expansion.
● Calcium sulphate dihydrate. The addition of a small amount of calcium sulphate dihydrate will also provide additional sites for nucleation.
(c) By carefully regulating the amount of the above additives, gypsum-based products can be produced with the correct degree of expansion appropriate to their application. Typically, the setting expansion for gypsum products is as follows:
Plaster 0.20–0.30 %

Stone 0.08–0.10 %
Densite 0.05–0.07 %

The slight setting expansion of stone and densite makes these materials ideal for the production of dies and casts for metal and ceramic work, where a high degree of accuracy is desirable. It is preferable for the cast to be slightly larger than the teeth.

When mixed with silica, the setting expansion of stone is considerably higher – typically 0.4% compared with 0.1% when used alone. Such gypsum-bonded investments are used for casting alloys with melting ranges below 1,000°C. The setting expansion enlarges the mould and helps to compensate for the contraction of the alloy on cooling. A special case is hygroscopic expansion, where the setting expansion of a gypsum-bonded investment material can be substantially increased to greater than 1.0% by immersing the material in water while it is setting. In air, the crystals tend to be drawn together due to the surface-tension effect of the water as the amount of free water reduces, thereby limiting the ability of the crystals to grow. When immersed in water the crystals can grow more freely, resulting in a greater degree of expansion.

See also **18**.

5 Healing abutments are used in preference to conventional implant abutments: (i) when it is difficult to assess the ultimate thickness of the soft tissue that is likely to exist after healing is complete following the second stage operation; (ii) when it is intended to use an angled or conical abutment.

6 (a) Denture-induced sore mouth, denture-associated stomatitis, or chronic atrophic candidosis from *Candida* species, usually *albicans*.
(b) Diabetes, iron-deficiency anaemia, steroid and antibiotic therapy and immunocompromising conditions.
(c) Immerse the denture each night in 2% hypochlorite solution until the red appearance is eliminated and the candidal infection has been resolved. Subsequently, ensure that adequate denture hygiene procedures are adopted.

See also **59**, **154** and **194**.

7 The alloy has the typical high strength properties of a Type IV gold alloy. The melting range, which consists of the solidus and liquidus temperatures, is useful in the selection of solders and casting investments. The liquidus temperature indicates the point at which the alloy becomes completely molten but the casting temperature will need to be higher than this. Liquidus temperatures under 1,000°C indicate that gypsum-bonded investment materials can be used safely.

Vickers hardness indicates the likely ability of a casting to resist abrasive wear and scratching, and to retain its polish. Tensile strength indicates the maximum stress that a structure can withstand before fracture in tension. Yield strength, which is closely comparable with elastic limit and proportional limit, represents the stress at which permanent deformation of the casting begins.

High tensile and yield strengths are desirable where stresses are expected to be high, such as with implant-supported frameworks, bridges, major connectors and clasps. Elongation is an indicator of ductility and values lower than 2–3% may indicate brittleness. The designations 's' and 'h' represent the alloy's softened and hardened states respectively. Note the substantial increases in surface hardness, and tensile and yield strengths following heat-treatment strengthening, also the essential need for such treatment if Type IV properties are to be fully obtained.

See also **100**.

8 (a) Spring cantilever bridge.
(b) The patient has failed to maintain adequate plaque control and this has led to marked inflammation. Compressive loading of the bar by occlusal action on the incisor pontic has grooved the mucosa of the palate.

9 Although the residual ridges appear to be favourable, it is evident that there has been some enlargement of the tongue such that it encroaches into the denture space. The design of the dentures is, therefore, likely to be compromised, making it difficult to achieve satisfactory tooth relationships consistent with good function. Even if the clinical situation were favourable, the fact that this patient has not satisfactorily worn complete dentures should indicate potential difficulties. He should be reminded of the limitations of treatment at the outset and not given false hope.

10 (a) First and second premolars and first molars only in each quadrant. No teeth should be placed on the sloping second/third molar mandibular region as this would induce instability by pushing the lower denture forwards down the slope during masticatory function.
(b) The central fossae of the mandibular teeth should always be placed over the centre of the ridge. The lower molars should be positioned over the lowest, flattest part of the ridge, must not encroach on to the posterior sloping region, and should be placed at right angles to the ridge. The premolar teeth should be positioned next so that they follow the curve of the ridge as it moves up towards the anterior region and away from the lowest (molar) region, and should also be at right angles to the ridge. This allows masticatory loads to be directed at right angles to the ridge, irrespective of the curve

of the ridge. In cases where mandibular denture stability is the major problem, it is advisable to set the lower teeth first in this way, with the uppers conforming to the lowers.

(c) A reduction in the buccolingual width of the posterior teeth will enable them to perform masticatory functions more efficiently, thereby preventing greater compressive forces (as with large molar teeth) being transmitted to the underlying tissue and bone. The use of all premolar teeth in the posterior regions, instead of molars, would have a similar effect in reducing transmitted forces. This is an important point to bear in mind when constructing dentures for patients with poor tissues and thin, sharp bone.

11 (a) Porosity – there are 3 main types that can occur during the processing of acrylic resin.

(i) Granular porosity. Incomplete mixing or wetting of the polymer powder particles by the monomer liquid produces a granular, dry mix, this giving a porous-like effect in the resin. It is therefore important to ensure complete wetting of the polymer by the monomer but with no undue excess monomer left over.

(ii) Contraction porosity. An excess of acrylic resin is needed within the packed flask in order to create pressure so that air voids can collapse (under spring pressure) and be replaced by the excess resin. Insufficient resin or insufficient pressure exerted on the flask during curing could lead to porosity voids being distributed throughout the entire resin denture.

(iii) Gaseous porosity. When the flask is filled with acrylic resin and closed together under spring pressure, the resin is ready to be processed or cured. This is normally achieved by placing the flask and spring clamp into a water or hot air bath. When selecting a curing cycle it is important to remember the following points:

• The polymerisation reaction is highly exothermic.

• The boiling point of the monomer is 100.3°C. If the resin temperature is allowed to go beyond this the monomer will boil, producing round voids at the hottest part of the resin. More monomer is found in the thickest areas and this is where gaseous porosity is usually seen.

• A popular and safe curing cycle is to heat the flask and resin to 70°C for 5–7 hours, followed by 2.5–3 hours at 100°C. Nearly all the conversion of monomer to polymer occurs at the 70°C temperature, during which time the exothermic reaction takes place. Although the resin temperature can approach 100°C, the likelihood of it exceeding the boiling temperature is diminished. The final cycle at 100°C should ensure that all the monomer is converted to polymer, especially in the thinner areas where the effect of exothermic heat is less severe.

(b) As the excess acrylic resin exits between the 2 halves of the flask as they are closed together, the 'flash' trapped causes an inevitable increase in vertical dimension. The cumulative increase of both maxillary and mandibular dentures can range from 1mm to 3mm, severely reducing the patient's free-way space. In order to correct this error, the maxillary and mandibular casts must have been mounted on to the articulator using a 'split cast' mounting technique. The processed dentures, still on the casts, can then be repositioned on to the articulator and the teeth adjusted.

See also **48** and **175**.

12 (a) The pain is caused by a chronic denture-induced ulcer which has a slightly hyperplastic buccal margin.
(b) The ulcer is deep, has been present for some weeks, and has become infected.
(c) Close examination indicates that this denture is not new and, therefore, the ulcer is caused by an alteration in the relationship between the right buccal flange and the peripheral soft tissues because of resorption of the lower alveolar ridge.

It is essential to remove the trauma immediately by either modifying the flange appropriately or, if this is not possible, asking the patient not to wear the lower denture.

When the ulcer and the lymph node have resolved, the management may be as follows:
● If the dentures are otherwise satisfactory the patient may be reassured and advised to continue with the denture.
● If the ulceration has become more frequent then a rebase of the denture is indicated if all other design factors are correct.
● If, however, the denture is not otherwise satisfactory, then a replacement should be considered.

See also **86**, **133** and **192**.

13 Where it is necessary for the crown of an artificial tooth to appear to emerge from normal gingivae, the contour of the crown or emergence profile must be related carefully to the soft tissue. The material illustrated in the question enables the soft tissue to be simulated.

14 (a) Parallel surfaces have been prepared on the crowns with a laboratory milling machine. The prepared surfaces extend lingually from a mesial proximal wall to a distal wall. The proximal surfaces are dished to create lateral resistance form and the gingival floors are well defined as a shoulder around the crowns. Proximal contacts between the crowns are displaced buccally to maintain horizontal stability.
(b) Milled crowns may be used to support and retain removable prostheses. In this case the crowns were used to support, retain and prevent rotation of a removable chrome-cobalt anterior saddle partial denture, thereby avoiding the use of unsightly clasps.

(c)As in all partial denture cases, the design should be planned as early as possible during treatment. Mounted study casts will highlight problems in connection with a design and may be used to construct a wax up of the finished case. Study preparations cut on a duplicate study cast will guide final tooth preparation. A large amount of tooth substance has to be removed to give sufficient room for milled crowns. Tooth preparation must follow the contours of the final crowns, leaving room for channels, boxes and occlusal rests. Deep preparations carry the risk of pulp exposure, a condition made less likely if radiographs are studied carefully to determine alignment of the anatomical crowns over the roots and the extent of the pulp chamber.

15 (a) (i) Poor ridge height, giving little support to the lower prosthesis.
(ii) Incorrect positioning and width of teeth.
(iii) Unsatisfactory occlusion.
(iv) Incorrect extension of the periphery.
(v) Poor fit of the denture base.
(vi) Overbuilt polished surface contours.
(b) Stability of the lower denture should be assessed at rest and with the mouth open. Displacement at rest usually indicates over-extension of the denture periphery or poor polished-surface contour. The effect of tongue movements, speech and swallowing should be observed. Displacement under these circumstances may indicate poor tooth position, inadequate fit of the denture base, or overbuilt polished surface contours. Minimal tooth contacts in intercuspal position and displacement during lateral excursions may indicate unsatisfactory occlusion. The position of the tongue and cheeks at rest should be determined, both with and without the lower denture present. Ease of movement of the denture while pressing on the ridge indicates unsatisfactory adaptation of the denture base.
(c) If the upper denture, tooth position, occlusion and vertical dimension are all satisfactory, adjustments to the periphery, polished surface contour and reline procedures can be undertaken on the existing denture. In all other circumstances a new denture should be constructed using appropriate techniques to prevent recurrence of the original problems.

16 (a) Two separate red and green thin occlusal test foils have been placed between the opposing teeth to mark tooth contacts in different mandibular positions. The coloured marks are well defined and are confined to a small area on each tooth because the foil is only 11μm thick. Left and right lateral excursions from the intercuspal position were recorded first using the green foil. Intercuspal (centric) contacts were then overlaid in red.
(b) The use of 2 different coloured test foils allows the operator to distinguish between contacts in intercuspal position and contacts made during lateral excursions. New restorations should be adjusted to conform to an

established intercuspal position using a single coloured foil. Once satisfactory intercuspal contacts are established, lateral excursion contacts should be assessed using another colour. Intercuspal contacts must be identified prior to adjustment of lateral interferences. This is achieved by overlaying the intercuspal contacts in a second colour after first indicating the lateral excursion contacts. Interferences in lateral excursions may then be removed. Guidance of the mandibular teeth is readily established using this technique to produce canine guided or group-function occlusion. Bilateral canine guidance has been established in this case.

17 (a) The neutral zone is the region that exists within the potential denture space, where the forces of the cheeks and lips balance those exerted by the tongue.
(b) Two basic techniques exist to record the neutral zone and to incorporate it into the denture design:
(i) A stable base with retention loops is loaded with impression material, a fluid material being preferred as the patient needs to be able to manipulate it easily. The patient is then instructed to make various exaggerated muscular facial movements, such as 'e' and 'o' sounds and touching the upper lip with the tip of the tongue. The resulting impression can then be duplicated and incorporated into the denture design.
(ii) The second method of recording the neutral zone is to load elastomeric-type impression material or disclosing paste on to the polished surfaces of the dentures at the try-in stage. The same movements and sounds are made as previously described. When the dentures are flasked, the new shape is incorporated into the plaster moulds.
   In both these cases, additions (under-extension) and trimming (over-extension) can be made until the denture/impression is stable during functional movements.
(c) A neutral-zone denture technique allows selected functional dynamic movement of the muscles to mould the impression material but does not allow it to fall on to and distort the lips, cheeks and tongue, as would be the case if the muscles were left passive. Patients therefore form the polished surface of the denture to take their own individual denture space shape. With the denture in place, the muscles of the lips, cheeks and tongue act against the denture to retain it against the denture-bearing areas even during exaggerated movements.
   See also **162**.

18 (a) Plaster. The dihydrate is heated in an open vessel and converted to hemihydrate, known as calcined calcium sulphate or β-hemihydrate. Dental stone. The dihydrate is heated under steam and pressure in an autoclave.

This autoclaved calcium sulphate is known as α-hemihydrate.

It should be noted that in both these cases the substance is chemically identical and only differs in form and structural detail.

(b) For plaster, the powder consists of large, irregular, porous particles. For dental stone, the powder consists of small, regular-shaped particles that are relatively non-porous.

(c) Plaster needs to be mixed with a large amount of water to obtain a satisfactory mix as much of the water is absorbed into the pores of the particles. The usual mix is 50ml of water for every 100g of powder.

Owing to the non-porous and regular structure of the stone particles, they can be packed more tightly together using less water. The mix is 25ml of water for every 100g of powder.

See also **4**.

19 The soft-tissue contour around an artificial crown may take several weeks to adjust to the morphology of the crown. Only when occlusal adjustments are complete and the soft tissue is stable should the final crown be constructed – provided that the patient's approval has been obtained.

20 (a) A single abutment tooth carrying a post with gold diaphragm, from which a screw-type stud attachment has been removed and replaced with a threaded-plastic transfer jig. There is also a carious root face present.

(b) The transfer jig is used to locate the exact relation of the attachment to the abutment and soft tissues. A silicone impression is used to record the soft tissues and the position of the T-shaped jig. The jig is unscrewed from the abutment tooth, attached to a dummy matrix and relocated in the impression before pouring the working cast. The overdenture may then be rebased and fitted with a new matrix cup. Before trying in the rebased denture a new stud of exactly the same type is screwed into the abutment tooth.

(c) It is essential to determine whether the stud requires a rigid or resilient attachment as the method of processing the denture in the laboratory differs depending on the type, and the fit of the denture will be affected.

21 This is an example of a Michigan- or Ramjford-type splint. It can be used at night by patients who are bruxists, as a mandibular repositioning device, or for the treatment of temporomandibular joint dysfunction problems. The hard acrylic resin has a flat occlusal surface in even contact with the opposing teeth, and with a canine rise built in for canine guidance.

See also **98**.

22 (a) There will be an increased masticatory load and, therefore, increased vertical and lateral forces on the overdenture. These will be transmitted to the abutment teeth and lead to further periodontal breakdown in the presence of established periodontal disease.

The increased load will also accelerate the alveolar bone resorption rate.

(b) (i) The denture base should be fully extended over the denture-bearing areas to reduce the adverse effect of the occlusal load. The occlusion should be planned to produce a functional balance in all excursions as far as possible to reduce the lateral loading on the alveolus, abutments and attachments.

(ii) The attachments may have to be placed slightly lingual to clear the overbite; this may compromise tongue space anteriorly.

(iii) An adequate interocclusal space should be provided to minimise occlusal load.

(c) Due to the increased alveolar resorption, more frequent relines will be necessary to maintain the fit of the denture and to reduce the load on the abutments by maintaining the appliance in the mucosa-borne mode.

See also **85, 95, 160, 165, 169** and **188**.

23 (a) An impression tray is a device into which a suitable material is inserted to make an impression. It is also used to carry, confine and control the impression. A properly formed tray should:

● Support the impression material in a predetermined contact with the oral tissues.

● Allow placement of pressure on selected areas of the denture bearing tissues while recording other areas in a nondisplaced state.

● Retain its shape through the impression procedure and pouring of the impression.

(b) The advantages of a special tray over a stock tray are:

● A more uniform thickness of impression material, giving greater accuracy with many materials.

● Easier location into and around the areas to be recorded.

● It can be designed so that more than 1 impression material can be used in the same tray where this technique is required.

● Special features can be more easily incorporated into special trays.

● Special trays can be constructed to carry any impression material the dentist may want to use.

(c) The determining factors in the type of special tray requested from the laboratory are:

● The types of ridge present – bony, undercut, flat and flabby.

● The types of tissue present – thick, uneven, compressible and tightly bound down.

- The type of impression material required to record accurately the conditions above.
- Whether the patient is dentate, partially dentate or edentulous.
- The type of appliance to be constructed from the impression.
  See also **190**.

24 (a) Infra bulge is the term used to describe a clasp that approaches the undercut from the gingival area of the tooth and is also commonly called a gingivally approaching clasp. Examples of infra-bulge clasps are Roach arms or I-bars.

Supra bulge is the term used to describe a clasp that approaches the undercut from the occlusal surface of the tooth and is also commonly called an occlusally approaching clasp. Examples of these are circumferential clasps, single arm clasps and 3-arm clasps.

(b) Major connectors can be divided as follows:
- Palatal plates and bars.
- Lingual plates and bars, sublingual bars, dental bars.
- Labial plates and bars.
- Palatal plates and bars can be subdivided into anterior, middle and posterior.

(c) Indirect retention can be described as follows. Ideally, a partial denture should be directly retained at all 4 corners of the arch. If, however, we have a Kennedy Class 1 situation, it will only be possible to clasp the 2 anterior corners. The free-end saddles will therefore be able to lift from the tissue and rotate around an axis formed by the clasps. Any element of the denture that is positioned on the opposite side of the rotational axis from the saddles, and which is firmly supported by the teeth, will resist movement of the saddles.

These elements of the denture do not directly help to retain the denture in place but 'indirectly' prevent removal of the denture when tipping of the denture occurs. Indirect retainers can take the form of occlusal and cingulum rests, claws, incisal rests, arms and parts of the connectors (both major and minor).

25 (i) Stock or factory made. These are horseshoe shapes of rubber or plastic. No modifications are possible in order to improve the fit. They are generally regarded as being unsatisfactory due to their poor fit and retention.

(ii) Mouth-fitted. There are 2 types of mouthguard that can be modified and fitted at the chairside:
- A thermoplastic shell, which is softened in hot water and then adapted to the teeth.

• A rubber or plastic shell, onto which a soft material is poured and allowed to set.
(iii) Laboratory made. These are made on articulated casts of the patient's teeth. There are 2 types:
• They are made by thermoforming polyvinyl/polyethylene blanks and are available in a range of colours.
• Alternatively, they are made from resilient silicone rubber by a flasking and packing technique.

26 (a) Acrylic resin denture base materials are usually supplied as a powder and liquid. The bulk of the powder is made up of polymer beads of polymethylmethacrylate, with diameters up to 100µm. These are produced by suspension polymerisation, where methylmethacrylate monomer plus initiator is suspended as droplets in a solution of starch or carboxymethylcellulose. The temperature is raised to decompose the peroxide and bring about polymerisation of the methylmethacrylate so that beads of polymethylmethacrylate are formed. The beads are then dried and will form a powder at room temperature.
(b) The benzoyl peroxide is the initiator.
(c) The salts of cadmium, iron or organic dyes are used as pigments to coat the clear beads and give them colour. Small fibres coated with pigment can also be added to give a veined appearance.
(d) The major component of the liquid is methylmethacrylate (mma) monomer. This is a clear liquid with a boiling point of 100.3°C, a high vapour pressure at room temperature, and a distinct odour.
    After mixing, the powder (polymer) and liquid (monomer) are polymerized using either heat or chemicals to form polymethylmethacrylate.
(e) Ethyleneglycoldimethacrylate is the cross-linking agent and is used to improve the physical properties of the set material. These agents are difunctional alkenes in which each of the 2 double bonds present is able to become polymerised into a separate chain, effectively linking 2 chains together.
(f) Hydroquinone is the inhibitor and is used to prolong the shelf-life of the liquid. Without an inhibitor, polymerisation of the monomer and cross-linking agent would occur slowly, even at room temperature.
(g) NN^1-dimethyl-P-toluidine is an activator and is found only in products that are called self-curing or cold-curing. The activator reacts with the benzoyl peroxide in the powder to create free radicals, these then initiate polymerization of the monomer.

27 (i) An upper 'spoon' denture of the type of design shown in **27A** is too small. The patient may swallow or inhale it.
(ii) The lower partial denture of the design shown in **27B**, known as the

'gum-stripper', has no rests to provide support. In the mandible, insufficient support is available from the mucosa and the gingivae is easily damaged. This might be considered an acceptable design for use as a temporary measure or as a transitional denture.

28 (a) The base of the denture is generally under-extended. This means that there is lack of peripheral support for the masticatory load, thus overloading the denture-bearing tissues over the alveolar ridge area. This increased masticatory load per unit of denture bearing mucoperiosteum usually results in generalised discomfort and pain.
(b) The main feature causing instability/looseness is the poor peripheral adaptation of the denture base to the surrounding musculature – sometimes referred to as lack of muscle balance.

29 (a) (i) Looseness and instability of both dentures.
(ii) Difficulty/inefficiency in eating.
(iii) Pain on the left side, particularly under the lower denture, due to the premature contact and overload on the mucoperiostium.
(b) It is probably caused by an error during the recording of centric jaw relationship when the rims would have been recorded with a premature contact on the right and lifted off the mucosa on the left. This error produces the opposite effect on the trial and finished dentures if undetected.
(c) The error is too great to be reduced by occlusal adjustment, so either a temporary occlusal veneer may be added or, preferably, the lower teeth should be removed, the occlusion re-recorded and the denture re-tried and finished.
    See also **106**, **110** and **174**.

30 It is essential that any superstructure attached to more than one implant imposes the minimum of lateral force when the prosthesis is permanently secured by screws to the abutment. It is therefore essential to provide the technician with transfer copings in an exact relationship to one another (and thus the abutments). Plaster is therefore a suitable impression material in this situation.

31 The bar has fractured through a weak soldered joint and may be repaired by re-soldering provided that the joint is strengthened.
    The fractured end of the bar is first ground away by approximately 0.20mm, before realigning and joining to the gold cylinder in the mouth using autopolymerising resin or hard wax. After investing in a soldering investment and removal of the resin or wax, the parts to be joined are then separated by a necessary small space into which new solder can flow. Before

re-soldering, a U-shaped piece of 1mm diameter round clasp wire is placed on the point of the bar that will be in contact with the gold cylinder. After soldering, the wire provides an enlarged and therefore stronger joint.

It is safe practice to wire-strengthen and re-solder any other weak joint at the same time. Depending on the manufacturer's recommendations, some bars require a strengthening heat treatment after soldering.

32 In excursive jaw movements with the teeth in contact, the path of the mandible is directed posteriorly by the movement of the condyles down their respective paths – in the rear of the mouth by the molar teeth, centrally by the premolars and in the front of the mouth by the movement of the lower incisor teeth against the inclines of the upper teeth.

Condylar path angles are determined from the patient's temporomandibular joints, while the setting of the posterior teeth and adjustment of the angle of incisal guidance is under the control of the prosthodontist or technician. Since incisal guidance is at the front of the articulator, it will have greatest influence on the angle of the contacting surfaces of the anterior teeth.

The ability of incisal guidance tables to establish a given incisal guidance angle provides a convenient substitute for the incisor teeth prior to their positioning in complete dentures. After all the teeth have been set to position, balanced occlusion and articulation should be checked on the articulator without mechanical incisal guidance.

See also **134**.

33 The defect is contraction porosity and occurs as cast molten metal cools and solidifies from a liquid to a solid state. More metal needs to be added during this stage and this is provided by using thicker sprues or bulkier reservoirs positioned on sprues close to the casting. Being of greater bulk than the casting, these parts remain molten for a longer period and can therefore supply further metal as required to the solidifying and contracting casting.

34 This patient's teeth are intrinsically discoloured through administration of tetracycline during development. Although the effects of tetracycline on the developing dentition are now well documented, there continues, nevertheless, to be a small number of individuals with this condition. Treatment depends upon the severity of the discoloration and level of patient concern. In severe cases it may be necessary to mask the discoloration with the placement of porcelain laminate veneers. Some judicious tooth preparation is desirable and, when combined with tints and modifiers beneath the veneers, aesthetics can be greatly improved. When the discoloration is particularly

severe and opaque veneers are used, teeth lose their vital appearance.
See also **140**.

35 There is maximum extension of the flanges of the saddle. The rest on the premolar is mesially placed. The part lingual plate will aid with indirect retention. A premolar denture tooth has been used instead of a second molar.

36 (a) The mental foveae (insertion of the mentalis muscles).
(b) Gradual resorption of non-functioning alveolar bone over a period of 12 years will cause the denture to be supported at its periphery only by those parts of the mandible that consist of basal bone that retains a function – in this case muscle insertions. Excess pressure then results in ulceration and pain.
(c) Relieve the denture over the ulcerated area to reduce inflammation and swelling before taking impressions. To prevent pressure recurring elsewhere, a temporary soft liner can be applied to the fitting surface of the lower denture.

37 Since the caries rate is low and the prognosis for retention of the teeth – other than the canines – is poor, the best form of treatment is probably an overdenture, retaining the lower canines as abutments. This can be achieved most easily by first making a transitional acrylic partial lower denture, to which the premolars and incisors can be incorporated by immediate addition. Later, after root filling the canines, their crowns can be removed and a further immediate addition made. The denture can later be replaced permanently.

38 (a) Loss of adequate posterior occlusion and a Class II division 2 occlusion has resulted in a deep overbite, traumatizing the palatal gingivae.
(b) The appliance is known as a Dahl appliance, after B. Dahl who first described the technique.
(c) The appliance is designed to increase the vertical dimension of the anterior teeth by providing a metal palatal bite plane, thus opening the posterior occlusion.
(d) The increased vertical dimension of the anterior teeth allows the posterior teeth to drift into occlusion by over-eruption or re-eruption. The anterior teeth may also be depressed, or a combination of these effects may occur. The net outcome is a change in the vertical relationship between the anterior and posterior teeth. In this case, the lower teeth are taken out of their traumatic occlusion with the upper soft tissues. The appliance may be used to create space in the anterior region prior to occlusal rehabilitation.

(e) The occlusion must be stabilised following successful tooth movement. This is achieved by making permanent additions to the palatal surfaces of the anterior teeth with, for example, resin-bonded castings or full coverage crowns. The posterior occlusion can then be stabilised as required with onlays, crowns and bridges.

39 An anterior horizontal reference point is being marked with the aid of a guide placed on the right lateral incisor. This point is used in conjunction with the posterior reference point (the tragus) to establish the horizontal reference plane (approximate to the Frankfort plane). The same guide is also used to assess the horizontal plane. The facebow records the relationship between the maxillary teeth and the condylar hinge axis in any position along the arc of the hinge axis. Incisal guidance provides the anterior determinant of movement, a feature independent of the horizontal plane; however the condylar guidance angle is directly related to the horizontal plane and provides the posterior determinants of movement.

It is essential to align the frame of the facebow with the horizontal reference and to use the same plane when measuring and recording condylar guidance angles. Excessive deviation of the facebow record from the correct horizontal plane will result in significant errors in the transfer of condylar guidance angles to the articulated casts. The cusp angles of restorations constructed on such casts may be too steep, causing posterior tooth interferences in lateral and protrusive movements.

40 Single tooth implants must be made well clear of the normal occlusion as all natural teeth are slightly intruded on biting. Osseointegrated implants are not intruded so much as a natural tooth. However, there is probably some minor movement of the bone around the implant, as well as an overall flexing of the jaw.

41 (a) The preliminary impression stage was omitted.
(b) Recording working impressions using stock trays is rarely satisfactory. This is because the trays do not extend in all regions to the full anatomical extent of the denture-bearing areas. This is particularly the case with the posterior border of the upper and the lingual extension of the lower – as illustrated in the photograph.
(c) The patient will usually complain of an upper denture which drops, and an unstable lower one which will probably also cause pain.

42 (i) Surveying.
(ii) Occlusal analysis.
(iii) Denture design.

(iv) Discussion with the patient.
(v) Construction of special trays.

43 No. The physiological movement of teeth means that the combination of implants and natural teeth in 1 fixed bridge will induce stresses on the bridge/implant interface, as well as the implant/bone interface. The support given to the bridge by the natural teeth should therefore be regarded as minimal.

44 (a) The attachments shown are extracoronal resilient ball-and-socket types, designed to support and retain distal free end saddle removable dentures. This attachment enables the prosthesis to move vertically and rotate around a single plane of movement. When used together the plane of movement of both attachments should ideally be parallel.
(b) Where possible, the attachments should be placed in line with the mandibular ridge to direct rotational movement of the saddle on to the ridge. Where 2 contralateral attachments are used they should be located to allow a parallel path of rotation, with no more than 5° of deviation. There is excessive angulation in this case between 2 attachments with the same path of insertion. This permits pure vertical but no rotational movement.
(c) Repeated loading of the prosthesis would produce torquing forces on the attachments. The resultant splaying of the matrix components will produce rapid wear and loss of direct retention.

45 Wax wafer registrations are being made for right (**45A**) and left (**45B**) mandibular excursions. Mandibular side-shift occurs during translation of the condyles which is recorded by the wafers. When translated to an arcon articulator, the right side-excursion record facilitates adjustment of the medial wall of the orbiting left condylar fossa into contact with the condyle, thus setting the side-shift for that condyle. The left excursion record enables setting of the contralateral fossa medial wall in the same manner.

The degree of mandibular side-shift depends upon the extent of the movement of the orbiting condyle from its rest position, thus a record of side-shift is made for only 1 position along the path of movement. Side-shift is described as having immediate and progressive components. A single record is unable to record the entire path of movement, thus the records are of use only on semi-adjustable articulators where the morphology of the fossa medial wall is fixed and where its movement is limited. It is necessary to use a pantograph or electronic equivalent to trace the entire pattern of side-shift, then a fully adjustable articulator is required to reproduce this path of movement.

46 (a) The patient has large tuberosities.

(b) The tuberosities are large both vertically, producing difficulties in extending the denture base to its correct posterior limit due to probable contact with the retromolar pads, and horizontally, producing buccal undercuts that will require blocking out, resulting in poor adaptation of the denture flange and a food trap.

(c) The only satisfactory way of overcoming the problems is to reduce the tuberosities surgically in both dimensions using a clear surgical template. This will ensure correct functional morphology on which to support and retain satisfactory dentures.

See also **153**.

47 Graph **47A** – flexible and resilient.
Graph **47B** – rigid, strong, ductile and tough.
Graph **47C** – rigid, weak and brittle.
Graph **47D** – flexible, weak and brittle.

48 (a) The denture is porous.

(b) See answer to **11(a)**.

(c) The denture cannot be polished and is liable to discolouration and fracture.

See also **11** and **175**.

49 There has been considerable resorption of the maxilla, such that the residual ridge is extremely atrophic. There is some erythema anteriorly, which may indicate that the tissues are being traumatised. Some denture-related hyperplasia is also evident to the right of the mid-line. Palpation of the edentulous ridge would almost certainly reveal it to be flabby and displaceable.

A flabby anterior ridge is usually associated with the presence of natural lower anterior teeth and absence of lower posterior teeth. Where a lower partial denture is not worn, forces on the upper denture are thought to accelerate the resorptive process, such that the anterior maxilla becomes flabby and the traumatised tissues erythematous. A lack of balancing contact posteriorly means that when the lower incisors contact the upper denture it tips, breaking the posterior seal so that the denture falls. Movement of the denture base further traumatises the anterior maxilla to compound the situation. In the presence of a full complement of natural lower teeth, trauma is inevitable and may also indicate a parafunctional habit.

There are 2 schools of thought with regard to impression techniques: mucostatic and mucocompressive. The former believe that a retentive denture can only be provided by recording the tissues in their undisturbed state.

The disadvantage of this is that pressure spots often result when the denture is loaded because of the uneven thickness of mucosa and irregularities in underlying bony architecture. The latter believe that it is more important to provide good support under load and hence favour a mucocompressive technique. The denture is, therefore, likely to be well supported when loaded but patients may complain that it is loose at rest because it does not fit the resting tissues but only the tissues under compression.

See also **94** and **148**.

50 (a) The lower illustration shows a single-arm clasp, with the retentive tip pointing towards the saddle. As the saddle lifts away from the tissue, the clasp tip is activated and forced to move up over the undercut, thereby resisting lifting of the saddle. The upper illustration shows the clasp tip pointing away from the saddle. As the saddle lifts, the retentive tip of the clasp moves downwards away from contact with the tooth and towards the tissue. The clasp is not activated and does not resist saddle movement.

If the undercuts that are present allow it, clasp tips should always point towards the free-end saddles. If the undercuts are not favourable, a recurved clasp may be used.

(b) Partial dentures with distal extensions will always rotate around a central axis. This is usually around a line drawn between the teeth that have been clasped (direct retainers). It is therefore better to place occlusal rests away from the saddles, on the other side of the rotational axis of the denture. For the saddles to lift, the rests would have to move downwards but they are prevented from doing so by the teeth on which they rest. This is called 'indirect retention' and is a very important secondary function of occlusal rests.

(c) The Roach clasp or I-bar tends to be fairly long and is used mainly on canines or premolars. As a consequence, it is frequently used to remove the denture by the patient. If this type of clasp is constructed in wrought metal it would be too flexible and would distort easily. A cast alloy, which tends to be more rigid – such as gold or cobalt chromium – would be preferable, the extra length of the clasp allowing enough flexure to move in and out of the undercuts.

51 (a) A metal framework is necessary to provide a strengthening reinforcement within an otherwise all-resin prosthesis. The framework also joins the implants together, with the intention of distributing occlusal loads as widely as possible over them. When such loads are contained within the strength of the implants and the physiological tolerance of their bone bed, this stress distribution may be thought of as providing safe bearing.

(b) Upon tightening the screws when placed in the mouth, a distorted prosthesis can deceive by straightening sufficiently to give the appearance of a correct fitting. Under these conditions some implants will be subject to a continuous tensile stress, while others will be under compression depending on their position and the nature of the framework distortion. Depending on their severity, such stresses are known to produce accelerated bone loss.

52 (a) The elastomeric impression materials are characterised by the fact that they are polymers that are used at a temperature above their glass transition temperature (Tg). The higher their temperature above the glass transition temperature, the more fluid these materials will be. The viscosity of the polymers used for impression materials is governed primarily by the molecular weight of the polymer (in other words, the length of the polymer chains) and the presence of additives such as fillers.
(b) The process that converts the liquid polymer to a solid is known as cross-linking. This involves a chemical reaction that binds the polymer chains together to form a 3-dimensional network structure. The setting reaction is via a platinum catalyst and a silanol. An important feature of this particular setting reaction is that there is no by-product.
(c) Addition-cured silicone impression materials have time-dependent properties and are classed as viscoelastic materials; that is they have properties similar to both liquids and solids. Owing to the viscous component, if put under load for any length of time the material will flow, thereby causing a permanent deformation and consequently a distortion of the impression. The viscous response can be minimised by rapid loading and unloading. The material will then tend to respond elastically – hence the short, sharp tug.

53 (a) Since alginate impression materials suffer from imbibition, the impression is likely to swell if left immersed in a liquid disinfectant for any length of time.
(b) The current recommendation is to use a proprietary disinfectant spray, and to leave the impression in a sealed bag for a disinfection time of 30 minutes.

See also **99**.

54 Although several options are possible, one that gives good results with minimal 'correction' is the double-pour Duralay[1] technique. When the fractured tooth has been prepared for a crown, insert the denture and make an impression of the preparation and seated denture *in situ* (ensure denture

---

[1] Reliance Dental Manufacturing Company, Worth, Illinois, USA.

does not tilt). When the impression material has set, remove the impression and ensure the margins are satisfactory. Next, take an impression of the opposing arch and record intermaxillary relations and shade. Now remove the denture and pour Duralay into the space created by the denture adjacent to the prepared tooth – the Duralay effectively replaces the denture. The master cast is then poured and the crown may be constructed using the Duralay clasp assembly as a guide.

55 This situation is often referred to as the 'combination syndrome', and may cause problems to both patient and practitioner. Care should be taken to ensure maximal peripheral seal and appropriately prescribed occlusal planes. While balanced articulation is probably impossible here, it is essential to reduce displacing forces as much as possible; occlusal balance in retruded contact position is essential. In addition, displacing contacts in functional excursions must be eliminated if the patient is to gain proficient control of his/her denture. Minor adjustments may be accomplished in a co-operative patient via selective grinding following location of prematurities with articulating paper (this may not be wholly reliable), or by asking the patient to self-grind using carborundum paste.

Another option, producing more a customised occlusion, is to take a face-bow transfer at the trial denture visit, in addition to a precentric occlusal record plus protrusive and right and left lateral records. A semi-adjustable articulator may be set in accordance with the patient's records, and the occlusion adjusted accordingly prior to finishing the denture.

See also **106**, **110** and **174**.

56 The amount of tooth exposure varies with the age of the subject. If the patient is in his/her early twenties it may easily be in excess of 4mm, an exposure that usually declines gradually to total concealment at about 55 years of age. This reduction is mainly due to a loss of tone in the tissues forming the face, with tooth wear having a reduced effect. As age increases the process continues, with greater concealment of the upper teeth and lower teeth being increasingly seen when the lips are parted. The upper teeth are only seen during smiling.

Owing to the natural processes of reducing upper tooth exposure in natural teeth, the amount of anterior tooth revealed by prostheses can strongly suggest maturity or youth.

57 (a) The fitting surfaces of castings are usually ground in an attempt to correct a misfitting to the die on which they were made. It will be noticed that ground areas are either dull or bright. Dull areas indicate that metal was removed before the porcelain was fired. Bright areas show that grinding was carried out after the addition of porcelain.

(b) The consequence of metal removal, especially when die-spacer coatings have been used, can mean that the restoration is retained largely by the cement and not the retentive form of the prepared tooth.

See also **149** and **191**.

58 Assuming the illustration depicts the clinical situation with the patient's mandible in the rest position, it is evident that there is a severe space limitation with very little resorption of the residual ridges. This may cause considerable difficulties in providing complete dentures and will affect the choice of denture teeth. The dentures will, therefore, have to be of an 'all acrylic design' and it may be necessary to leave the molar teeth off. The use of porcelain teeth in such a situation will not be possible, since porcelain posterior teeth have a mechanical interlock (diatoric) on their under-surface, which retains the tooth in the processed denture. In this case, it would not be possible to reduce porcelain teeth sufficiently for them to be accommodated and at the same time retain their mechanical interlock. Porcelain teeth can, therefore, only be used where there is an appropriate inter-ridge separation that is sufficient to allow for tooth and denture base material.

59 (a) The patient is allergic to nickel.

(b) Skin tests for contact sensitivity should be made. If confirmed as a nickel allergy, a denture must be made of a non-nickel alloy or have a polymeric base.

See also **6, 154** and **194**.

60 (a) Bleaching of the dentures is occurring. Either the denture cleanser contains hypochlorite or the dentures are being placed in an immersion cleaner for an excessive period of time at too high a temperature.

(b) The patient should be advised to either use a non-hypochlorite denture cleanser or follow the manufacturer's instructions carefully.

See also **121** and **198**.

61 The arch form is considerably distorted because of the loss of some posterior teeth and wear affecting the anteriors. The cause of the wear should be established. In this case, the large slide from RCP to ICP coupled with a high intake of natural fruit juice has combined to produce significant tooth wear. Assessment of tooth position and vertical dimension in retruded contact position should be made when considering a treatment plan.

● Give dietary advice relating to citrus fruit erosion.
● Construct a splint to establish occlusion in RCP.

- Assess tolerance of the splint and resolution of TMJ symptoms.
- Make a diagnostic wax-up of the repositioned and reorganised occlusion.
- Provide an orthodonic appliance to move the anterior teeth forward to gain anterior tooth stability.
- Construct crowns and bridges on the repositioned teeth to the new vertical dimension, thus establishing a stable anterior and posterior occlusion.

62 The advantages are the ease of removal and the transfer of functional loading via a metal-to-metal contact. However, cemented crowns and small bridges benefit aesthetically from the absence of screw access holes. The use of temporary cement allows removal of the crown or bridge with conventional removal devices. It is important to have the ability to access and, if necessary, treat an individual implant/abutment unit.

63 (a) The patient complained that the denture was loose and dropped down at the back.
(b) The original posterior border of the denture may be seen showing through the rebase impression. This indicates marked under-extension of the border, with a consequent lack of peripheral seal.
(c) All undercuts are removed, the borders are corrected using green-stick composition and the posterior border is extended carefully using impression compound, ensuring good support for the zinc oxide impression material.

64 When the metal is removed from the investment following casting, it may be electrolytically polished. Several types of electrolyte are available but a common one is based on phosphoric acid and glycerin. The fitting surfaces of the denture must be protected with a coating of wax or varnish. Immersion should be for about 10 minutes with a current of approximately 3A at 6V. The casting may be tried in the mouth following this stage.
  Further polishing is achieved mechanically. The first stage uses a rubber wheel impregnated with an abrasive agent. The second stage is to polish the surface using a felt wheel or bristle brush and a proprietary polishing block.
  Final cleaning in an ultrasonic bath or in a detergent solution removes grease and dirt.

65 This is a silicone impression taken in a stock tray. The dual viscosity, single stage technique was used, whereby a light-bodied material was syringed around the abutment teeth while a heavy-bodied material was placed in the tray. Both viscosities must flow together before setting, and an addition-cured silicone is to be preferred when using a stock tray.

66 (a) The dentine and enamel shade porcelains are essentially feldspathic glasses. In contrast, the opaque porcelain consists of a feldspathic glass with up to 40–50% polycrystalline alumina. The alumina particles are much stronger than the glass and are more effective at preventing crack propagation. While the flexural strength of feldspathic porcelain is approximately 60MPa, this is raised to 120–80MPa for the aluminous porcelains and represents a 2- to 3-fold increase in the strength of a porcelain jacket crown.
(b) Although the compressive strength of dental porcelain is high (350–550MPa), its tensile strength is very low (20–40MPa). Being a glass, the material lacks any fracture toughness. The maximum strain that a glass can withstand is less than 0.1%. The material is extremely sensitive to the presence of surface micro-cracks and this represents one of the major drawbacks in the use of porcelain.

On cooling from the furnace, the outside of the porcelain will cool more rapidly than the interior, especially since the porcelain has a low thermal conductivity. This means that the outside surface initially contracts more, such that on further cooling there is a compressive load on the outside and a residual tensile stress on the inside surface as the interior is prevented from shrinking by the outside skin. If the differential dimensional change is sufficient, the internal surface layer under tension will rupture to relieve the stresses. Thus the internal surface will contain a large number of minute cracks and it is these that will ultimately cause the crown to fracture catastrophically.

67 (a) Since the internal fitting surface is the most likely source of fracture of a crown, the replacement of a core porcelain with a metal will provide a substantial improvement. This is because metals have an inherent fracture toughness and are therefore considerably less prone to fracture. In fact, metals tend to fail by permanent deformation when their yield strength is exceeded. This is unlikely to happen under normal occlusal loadings.
(b) One of the most likely modes of failure with the metal–ceramic system is the separation of the porcelain from the metal due to an interfacial breakdown. Thus the success of the system depends on the quality of the bond between the metal and the ceramic.

68 Since there is often a considerable loss of labial and buccal alveolar bone in the upper jaw, the position of the artificial teeth must often be at some distance from their support. Removable prostheses attached to a sub-frame by clips allow good soft-tissue support, more freedom in the positioning of artificial teeth and easier cleaning of both the substructure and the prosthesis in comparison with a fixed prosthesis.

69 (a) The tongue space has been cramped, particularly on the left side, by placing the posterior teeth too far lingually and thus causing instability. Additionally, the occlusal table (posterior tooth width) is too great, thereby compounding the cramped tongue space.

(b) A narrower mould of posterior teeth has been selected to allow maximum tongue space, and these have been set carefully in the denture space (zone of minimal conflict) between the lingual and buccal tissues to gain maximum stability of the denture.

See also **180**.

70 While it is true that most patients manage with prostheses made on hinge articulators, the wearers must change the way they eat in order to accommodate their imbalanced dentures. When this accommodation cannot be made satisfactorily, cuspal interferences cause denture movements that in turn produce pain and discomfort to the wearer.

Providing that they are correctly programmed, adjustable articulators may be used to obtain occlusal balance between the teeth and so reduce denture-displacing movements. However, such articulators and the technique for using them are highly user-sensitive. There is no advantage at all to using articulators, however refined, if they are used in the same way as hinge articulators.

Although the natural teeth in most mouths have gross cuspal interferences, they are securely supported in bone; this is not the case with mucosal-supported complete dentures.

71 (a) A short root containing a small post with circumferential bone loss extending between the proximal alveolar crests and around the root apex of the left lateral incisor. The tooth, and consequently the bridge, is likely to have a hopeless prognosis.

(b) The left anterior bridge will require removal in order to extract the remnants of the left lateral incisor root. A temporary removable acrylic partial denture is required before proceeding with one of the following:

- A removable partial denture in metal or acrylic.
- A new fixed-fixed anterior bridge involving all anterior teeth, including the first premolars as additional abutments.
- An attachment-retained removable partial denture.
- Single-unit osseointegrated implants.

72 (a) The attempt to give the patient the appearance she requested has resulted in a reduced anterior overjet and nipping of the lip at the contact of the incisal edges of the maxillary and mandibular anterior teeth.

(b) Increase the overjet by reducing the labial surface of the lower incisors, but only if this can be done without detriment to the appearance. Otherwise, a new lower denture must be made with repositioned lower incisors.

73 (a) If the dentures are designed correctly this patient had a Class II division I incisor relationship on a Class II base.

(b) The anterior teeth must be set in a similar Class II incisor relationship, the uppers to support the lip in its original position, and the lowers with their necks on the ridge and slightly proclined to provide a harmonious and stable relationship with the active lower lip. This not only provides stable dentures but also restores the profile and aesthetics.

(c) No. A balanced occlusion is not achieved in protrusion because the overjet has to be too great, moreover, these patients normally use a vertical action to chew rather than a slide.

74 Rubbing alginate impression material over the occlusal and incisal surfaces of the teeth prior to inserting the impression tray. This eliminates air blows which can cause errors in the occlusion of the casts.

75 (a) Elemental metals are not generally useful because of limitations in their properties. Most metals in common use are a mixture of two or more metallic elements or even non-metals. They are usually produced by fusion of the elements above their melting temperature. Such a solid mixture of two or more metals or metalloids is called an alloy.

(b) A phase is defined as a structurally homogeneous part of the system that is separated from other parts by a definite physical boundary. Each phase will have its own distinct structure and associated properties. The commonly cited phases are the gas, liquid and solid phases as these are markedly different from one another. A substance can include several phases. For example, water would be considered a single-phase structure, whereas a mixture of water and oil would consist of two phases. Sand, on the other hand, would be considered a single-phase system even though it is made up of lots of individual particles, since each particle of sand is identical. A phase may have more than 1 component – for example, saline, an aqueous solution of sodium chloride and water.

(c) When two metallic elements are dissolved into one another, a solid solution is formed. A solid solution is a mixture of elements at the atomic level and is analogous to a mixture of liquids that are soluble in one another. There are two types of solid solutions: substitutional and interstitial.

76 This is usually pathognomonic of the denture base interfering with the movement of the coronoid process and can be determined by palpation of the patient's coronoid process with the dentures out and on wide opening. It is also diagnosed by a characteristic wipe-off when pressure-relief paste is used.

77 This is a bar unit. While this overdenture preserves alveolar bone, the patient must be made aware of the need to maintain thorough oral hygiene and denture hygiene. The need for additional stability and retention are obvious factors in the selection of this type of attachment and the abutment teeth should be almost parallel. The bar should not be cantilevered more than 4mm anterior to the abutment teeth and sufficient height of abutment is required to facilitate flossing under the bar. A trial set-up is required to ensure that sufficient space exists, both anteroposteriorly and vertically for the bar assembly, otherwise speech problems may arise.

78 There is clear evidence of marked facetting of the denture teeth. This should warn that the patient has a parafunctional habit and, upon questioning, he/she may admit to nocturnal bruxism or clenching. In a case such as this, it is important to establish that the design of the dentures is satisfactory in terms of occlusion and, more importantly, occlusal vertical dimension. Assuming a satisfactory design, the patient should be encouraged to leave the dentures out at night.

79 The device is a tooth undercut measuring gauge. Placed against the tooth that is required to be clasped, a shank contacts at the survey line with a horizontal spur of metal adjusted until it also contacts the tooth. The projection of this spur indicates the amount of tooth undercut present, measured in millimetres. The tip of a retentive clasp arm will contact a tooth in a measured undercut appropriate for the following conditions:
- Size of the tooth.
- Bone support of the tooth.
- Modulus of elasticity of the alloy used to make the clasp arm.
- Angle of approach of the arm to the tooth.
- Cross-section, length and taper of the arm.
  See also **3, 186, 193** and **200**.

80 (a) A post-normal occlusion has been achieved – in other words, the lower teeth are at least half a unit behind the uppers. This has most likely been caused by the clinician recording centric jaw relationship about half a unit in protrusion. The error then remained unnoticed at the assessment of the trial dentures and was reproduced in the finished complete dentures. This is one of the most common clinical errors in prosthodontics.
(b) This depends on the degree of error. Dentures with a small antero-posterior discrepancy in occlusion should preferably be mounted on an articulator using an accurate occlusal record, the occlusion corrected in the laboratory by adjustment and then the dentures polished and reinserted. If, however, the error is as large as illustrated, the above technique only serves to ruin the cuspal anatomy and remove any possible semblance of balanced occlusion that existed, thereby giving a poor result. Remake of the appropriate (usually lower) denture will be necessary in this case.

81 This is a case of enamel hypoplasia, often associated with a childhood illness. The disturbance in enamel formation gives rise to defects, which subsequently become stained. Characteristically, these defects form bands on the teeth, whose position is related to the timing of the disturbance relative to tooth development. In this case, the pits, after the teeth have been cleaned and the stain removed, could be restored by means of an adhesive filling material. Where hypoplasia is more generalised, porcelain laminate veneers may be the treatment of choice. Although in both cases it is important to remove all traces of stain thoroughly, it is especially important if porcelain veneers are used. In a case such as this, tooth shade is not being altered and, as translucent veneers would be indicated, the stain would almost certainly 'show through'.

82 (a) Fracture of ceramics generally occurs from a flaw at the free surface. Thus, if a free surface can be removed the potential for fracture is much reduced. In porcelain-jacket crowns, the fitting surface is, for all intents and purposes, a free surface, and any micro-cracks present on the surface are the source of catastrophic crack propagation. When a ceramic restoration is bonded to the underlying enamel or dentine using appropriate adhesive procedures, this free surface is effectively removed as the ceramic restoration has now become an integral part of the tooth structure. Consequently, this source of crack initiation has been eliminated and the ceramic is fully supported by the tooth tissues. Should this adhesive bond break down, the ceramic will eventually fracture.
(b) Ceramics for dentine-bonded crowns, veneers and inlays consist of feldspathic glasses with crystalline inclusions of leucite. There are also glass-ceramics which consist of a glass matrix with a crystalline phase such as flu-

oromica. The fitting surface of these ceramics is inherently rough due to the gritblasting process used to remove the refractory/investment. The application of hydrofluoric acid to the fitting surface of these ceramics enhances the surface roughness as it results in the preferential removal of either the crystalline phase or the glassy phase.

The surface of glass, being ionic in nature, readily absorbs water, forming a well-bonded surface layer of highly polar hydroxyl groups. A silane coupling agent, when applied to the glass, will displace the water on the surface and form a chemical bond with the ceramic. The function of the coupling agent is to provide a strong chemical link between the oxide groups on the glass surface and the polymer molecules of the resin. Thus a micromechanical bond is created by the gritblasting and etching procedures, and a chemical bond is formed by the application of a silane coupling agent.

83 (i) Inappropriate initial tightening. Each screw has an idiosyncratic/individual optimum torque. Depending on their surface finish, the consistency of the alloy of which they are made, the intrinsic design and the internal form and accuracy of the abutment screw thread, the torque of gold-alloy screws is between 10Ncm and 15Ncm.
(ii) An imperfect fit – either vertical or horizontal – between the bridge components and the abutments will prevent an adequate foreload being applied to the interface; this in turn will cause screw-loosening or premature fracture.
Note: Excessive functional loading is most unlikely to result in screw-loosening or fracture once the appropriate pre-load has been applied.
See also **176**.

84 (a) The pictures show that the mentalis muscles must be contracted powerfully to achieve lip contact, hence the occlusal face height is too great, the dentures lack freeway space and occlusal interference is causing denture instability. The prominence of the lower lip probably means that the lower denture teeth are sited too far labially, so adding to the instability of the lower denture.
(b) New complete dentures must be made with correct jaw relations and correctly sited teeth.

85 (a) Chronic marginal gingivitis is present around the tooth crowns and root faces. Early signs of caries are visible on the palatal aspect of the upper right canine root.
(b) The patient has been provided with an overdenture prosthesis to replace the missing and root-filled anterior teeth. Failure to remove plaque from the prosthesis and the overdenture abutments has caused a local inflammatory

response in the neighbouring soft tissues. Failure to relieve acrylic surrounding the gingival margins of the abutments has allowed mechanical action to enhance the irritation of the plaque in these areas.

(c) (i) Plaque on the teeth and prosthesis should be disclosed with a suitable solution. The accumulations should be shown to the patient as part of routine oral-hygiene instruction.

(ii) Dietary advice should be given on the frequency and quantity of sugar intake.

(iii) Antiseptic and fluoride mouthwash should be prescribed until the next review appointment.

(iv) Acrylic contacting the soft tissue surrounding the root-face abutments should be relieved.

See also **22, 95, 160, 165, 169** and **188**.

86 Although the appearance of the ulcer resembles that of a large denture ulcer, the associated white patches and the lymph node enlargement are suspicious and warrant extra care. The denture should be relieved over the area of the ulcer and, if necessary, a soft lining material should be applied to relieve pain and an antiseptic mouthwash prescribed to eliminate secondary infection. Review a week later and if the appearance is unchanged the patient should be referred urgently to an oral surgeon so that a diagnosis of malignancy can be excluded.

See also **12, 133** and **192**.

87 (i) All screws stretch slightly on being tightened. To ensure that the optimum pre-load is applied to the abutment/fixture interface, it is essential that the optimum torque is applied to the abutment screw.

(ii) During the tightening process, the asperities on the surface of the internal and external screw threads become flattened, leading to a diminution of the force being applied to the abutment/fixture interface.

(iii) When a healing cap is removed from the head of an abutment, some of the reverse torque is transmitted to the abutment screw – fixture interface. This slight loosening must be eliminated by retightening the abutment screw.

88 The patient has a neglected dentition and a Class III skeletal pattern with incisor teeth in an edge-to-edge relationship. There are standing molar teeth that maintain the occlusal vertical dimension.

Some residual roots can usefully be removed at this stage, as can gross calculus accretions. Owing to the presence of occlusal and incisal stops, registration and denture construction is greatly facilitated. The main problem is likely to be related to the skeletal relationship and the apparent arch discrepancy, in that the maxilla appears to be somewhat narrower than the mandible. This will compromise tooth position and it may be necessary to set the posterior teeth in a crossbite. Although some patients in a situation such as this would wish to see the denture teeth placed in a more 'natural relationship', expections should not be raised, since this would not be possible without surgery to correct the skeletal disproportion. With time and continual resorption, stability of the upper denture often becomes a problem due to forward placement of the upper anterior teeth relative to the residual ridge and the cantilever effect that this produces.

89 (a) This is the swing-lock system. The retention system is based on a swinging labial bar which runs between the gingival margins and the labial sulcus. The bar is hinged at one side and locks at the other as the struts running vertically from the bar engage the cervical undercuts near the gingival margins of the anterior teeth. This provides a removable partial denture which is stable and well retained when the swinging bar is locked in the closed position.
(b) It is specifically designed for the lower distal extension saddle situation but it may also be used for the upper where conventional means of retaining removable partial dentures are not available. Classically this is found where only the lower anterior teeth are present and where there are no suitable undercuts for conventional clasps. In this situation, it also overcomes the problems of unsightly and sometimes uncomfortable conventional clasps related to the lower teeth.
(c) Where the patient has a low lip line or smile line, the cervical struts may be overlaid with a suitably tinted acrylic gingival veneer as illustrated in this case.
(d) The swing-lock denture, by virtue of its design, covers a large area of gingival tissues – and on the labial aspects in particular – when designed with the veneer. Patient selection is therefore very important and high standards of oral hygiene are mandatory.

90 The patient's right first premolar tooth has a clasp arm on its buccal surface, which is not reciprocated. The required toothborne saddle on the patient's left side is not provided with an occlusal rest on the first premolar tooth and the occlusal rest on the molar tooth is attached to a clasp part, which is flexible.
  A lack of reciprocation can result in lateral tooth movement from retentive arm tooth pressure on denture insertion and removal. Since the denture has a reduced area of coverage because of intended tooth support, the lack of adequate occlusal rests will allow the saddle to be depressed into the mucosa on this side.

91 (b) The permanent natural teeth of most subjects in all age groups usually follow the curve of the lower lip on smiling.

92 While no coverage is an option, most patients would wish to have an interim prosthesis for social reasons. Whichever option is selected, care must be taken to ensure that the implant fixture receives no loading during the healing phase (4–6 months in the maxilla). Toothborne dentures may be prescribed, as may etched restorations, although the latter may prove expensive temporary restorations. Vacuum-formed splints with tooth-coloured resin in the pontic area may be used, as may harder acrylic splints with full occlusal coverage; in both cases, care must be taken to ensure that the patient's occlusion is not disturbed.

A simple option is the so-called Manchester veneer: interproximal rests are placed on the abutment teeth and an impression is taken of the prepared teeth. The technician relieves the region of the implant with 0.5mm of tin foil and blocks out undercuts gingival to the interproximal rests prior to constructing a labial veneer incorporating an acrylic pontic.

93 (a) On the palate, just anterior to the vibrating line so that the posterior border of the denture lies on non-mobile tissues.
(b) The vibrating line is best marked on the mucosa with an indelible pencil, and then transferred during the recording of the impression or delineated by marking the corresponding position on the working cast.
(c) This is achieved by creating a rounded groove which runs from one hamular notch to the other just anterior to the post-dam line. It is created slightly deeper in the regions where the submucosa is thicker around the palatal vessels, and shallower where it is tightly bound down in the centre of the palate. When the denture is finished, this rounded ridge on the fitting surface ensures a good seal at the posterior border by displacing the tissues slightly.

94 (a) This is a fibrous and mobile (flabby) upper ridge. The alveolar bone has been replaced almost completely by fibrous tissue.
(b) The flabby ridge is normally caused by excessive loading on a complete upper denture which has been worn for many years and which is opposed by natural lower teeth. Classically, the condition is usually seen in the anterior region where the complete upper denture has been opposed by lower natural anterior teeth only; the partial lower denture will have been discarded by the patient long since.
(c) The main problem for the patient wearing a complete upper denture on such movable tissue is that the support is unstable and the denture tends to tip in function and become easily displaced. This support problem may be

reduced by using a differential-compression impression technique for recording the working impression. This minimises the amount of movement of the denture in function because the tissue is compressed but not displaced by the impression technique, so creating a more stable situation.

Surgical intervention using ridge augmentation and vestibuloplasty is rarely indicated as patients with this condition are often elderly and may also be medically compromised.

See also **49** and **148**.

95 (a) (i) The upper left central incisor has been devitalised, root-filled and a post and coping prepared on which to retain a precision attachment.
(ii) The upper right central incisor is vital and has been domed and polished; the cervical undercut has been removed.
(iii) The upper right lateral incisor has been devitalised and root-filled, the root face has been domed and an amalgam core has been inserted, the root face has been polished and the cervical undercuts removed.
(iv) The upper right canine has a similar preparation to the left central incisor, including root-canal filling and the preparation of a post and coping to retain a precision attachment. For both, the left central and right canine root anchors were selected for retainers.
(b) Apart from the anchors, which provide very positive retention, the peripheral seal derived from the fully extended complete upper base makes a useful contribution to the retention.

See also **22**, **85**, **160**, **165**, **169** and **188**.

96 (a) The Bonwill triangle is an equilateral triangle of approximately 100–110mm (depending on the make of the articulator used), measured from the tip of the incisal guidance pin of the articulator to both condyle heads of the articulator, and then between each condyle head. It is used as an average method of mounting casts (dentate or edentulous) onto an articulator.
(b) With the Bonwill triangle, an elastic band is placed around the notches provided on the rear pillars of the articulator, while at the front the elastic band is positioned to correspond to the incisal guidance pin. The maxillary and mandibular casts are then placed on pieces of plasticine, and these in turn are placed on the lower arm of the articulator and adjusted until the occlusal plane of the registration blocks/meeting of the natural teeth corresponds to the elastic band. The antero-posterior position of the casts should be adjusted so that the incisal guidance pin just touches the mesio-incisal angles of the upper maxillary incisors (lower incisors if the uppers are missing), or the junction of the centre-line and occlusal plane if registration blocks are on edentulous casts. The casts can then be attached to the upper and lower arms of the articulator with plaster, the upper cast being attached first.

The use of a facebow allows the relationship of upper and lower casts to be positioned within the articulator in exactly the same relationship to the articulator's condyle elements as the patient's upper and lower jaws (ridges or teeth) relate to their own condyle heads. With certain facebows it is also possible to measure the condylar angles, and again these can be transferred to the articulator.

If appliances are made on articulators where the casts are in the same relationship to the condyle heads as the patient's own anatomy, then a personalised accurate appliance can be made. With casts mounted in an average position on the articulator using an average condylar angle (30°), a compromised appliance will result, which the patient will have to 'wear in'. It is therefore preferable to use a facebow and to record condylar angle if personalised dentures are to be constructed.

97 Hypernasal speech in an adult patient with a cleft palate is something that cannot be corrected if it has been present since childhood and the patient's expectations should not be raised. Denture construction in such individuals is, in general, fairly straightforward, although care must be taken at the impression stage. A careful impression technique is required since materials can lodge in undercuts and cause trauma upon removal.

Where the cleft has been repaired, care should be taken to ensure that there are no residual fistulae, since extrusion of material up into the nasal floor is not uncommon and, once there, can be very difficult to remove. Small defects are often best packed with paraffin gauze prior to impression procedures, and care over the quantity and placement of material should then ensure that no mishaps occur. In a large, non-repaired cleft such as this, it is sometimes desirable to engage undercuts formed by the residual palatal shelves – dependent to some extent upon tissue quality and degree of displacability – by a denture extension. The correct amount of undercut is often best selected by blocking out unwanted undercut on the master-cast with plaster, prior to processing the final denture. Engaging too much undercut will cause trauma upon placement and removal of the denture which may necessitate some adjustment.

See also **141**.

98 It is evident that the 6 upper anterior crowns are failing. Porcelain has been lost from the incisal edges on the central incisors and left canine in particular. Around the lateral incisors and canines there is a marked chronic marginal gingivitis.

With such marked damage to metal-ceramic restorations and apparent flattening of the lower anterior teeth, it is evident that this patient must have a parafunctional habit. In such cases, the location of the metal–ceramic interface is crucial. Of particular importance is the position of opposing tooth contact in relation to the interface. In this case the metal–ceramic interface is near the incisal edge. The burnishing effect of the opposing tooth gliding across this junction causes metal creep and introduces stress at the metal–ceramic interface. Stresses are released when the porcelain flakes off the labial surface.

Treatment should aim at preventing further damage, which will require the patient to wear a nocturnal splint. Such splints should be constructed to avoid unwanted tooth movements. This requires contact of all opposing teeth at a slightly increased occlusal vertical dimension. An upper splint is generally preferable, being easier to construct so that it includes canine guidance, whereby posterior teeth disclude in lateral and protrusive excursions. The splint also prevents further damage and provides visible evidence of parafunctional activity (as the splint wears); in some individuals it may also help to break the parafunctional habit (see also **21**).

By careful design and, in particular, placement of the metal–ceramic junction, this problem can often be avoided. However, where a natural tooth occludes against porcelain, great care must be taken as wear of the opposing natural tooth may ensue if the porcelain surface is not properly glazed.

99 (a) The alginates are polymers based on alginic acid (derived from a marine plant) with a molecular weight of 20,000 to 200,000. When mixed with water, a sol–gel reaction occurs which cross-links the polymer chain and results in a 3-dimensional network structure. As this is an irreversible process the material can only be used once.

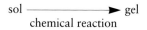

sol ———————→ gel
chemical reaction

(b) The dimensional stability of alginate impression materials can be affected in 1 of 2 ways, both being due to the water-based gel-like structure of these materials:
● Syneresis. This is where water is pushed out onto the surface of the impression as the gel molecules are drawn closer together, the driving force being built in stress and heat. The water then evaporates from the surface and causes the impression material to shrink.
● Imbibition. This is the uptake of water that occurs if the material has lost too much water, possibly as a result of inadequate storage technique. If this occurs, distortion of the impression will result as the internal stresses, which are always present, are relieved during the process.
(c) The impression must be rinsed after removal from the patient's mouth to remove any saliva (this will interfere with the setting of the gypsum cast).

Any surface water should be removed prior to pouring the cast. Residual water will dilute the cast material and will result in a soft surface that is easily damaged.

The alginate should not be left on the cast for too long as it becomes difficult to separate if allowed to dry out. This will result in a poor surface finish as bits of the alginate remain on the surface.

See also 53.

100 (a) ● The silver has a slight strengthening effect and counteracts the reddish appearance of the copper.
● The copper increases the strength and reduces the melting temperature. The limit to the amount of copper that can be added is 16% as amounts in excess of this tend to cause tarnishing of the alloy.
● Platinum increases the strength and the melting-point temperature.
● Palladium has the same effect as platinum but is considerably cheaper.
● Zinc acts as a scavenger during casting by preventing oxidation of the alloying elements. It also helps to improve the castability of the alloy.
(b) ● Type I alloys are best used for inlays in low-stress situations.
● Type II alloys can be used for most inlays except those with thin sections.
● Type III alloys can be used for all inlays, onlays, full-coverage crowns and bridges.
● Type IV alloys are used in partial denture construction, particularly clasp arms.
(c) The most effective strengthening mechanism for copper in gold is order hardening. This involves reheating the alloy to 400°C and holding it at that temperature for approximately 30 minutes. This hardening heat treatment is carried out after the homogenising anneal. Rather than being randomly distributed, the process causes the copper atoms to arrange themselves in little ordered clusters. This ordered structure has a lower internal energy than the disordered structure, and this has the effect of raising the yield stress and hardness of the alloy. For order hardening to occur there must be at least 11% copper in the gold alloy. Type I and Type II gold alloys have insufficient copper for this to happen. Type III gold alloys have just enough copper and a small improvement in strength is observed. With Type IV gold alloys, the improvement in strength is quite significant.

See also 7.

101 As with a post crown, the rotational forces imposed on the abutment screw must be resisted. It is therefore necessary to ensure that the abutment screw is tightened to the design torque. The physical properties of the gold-alloy screw allow a greater torque to be applied to the screw than if a screw made of pure titanium was used.

The sliding movement of titanium over titanium, as occurs when a conventional abutment screw is tightened into a fixture, is impeded by the surface characteristics of titanium. However, when a gold-alloy surface is in contact with a titanium surface there is less resistance and it is possible to apply higher torque without resulting in fracture.

102 (a) Excess freeway space or insufficient posterior overjet.
(b) If the cause is excess freeway space but the patient is otherwise satisfied with the dentures, encourage the patient to persevere in the hope that better muscle control will overcome the problem. If this fails, a new lower denture must be provided with less freeway space.

If the problem is one of insufficient posterior overjet, the overjet may be increased by reducing the buccal surfaces of the offending lower teeth. Always check that the traumatised tissue is related to opposing artificial teeth. If it is related to a contact between the denture base in the tuberosity and retromolar regions, the bases themselves must be thinned so that they are prevented from coming into contact with each other.

103 It is possible that the reline has increased the face height and reduced the freeway space but, in this case, the sensation is more likely to come from the lower denture-bearing area where the pressure is greater. From the picture it is more likely that the denture has been relined with an autopolymerizing resin, and that the symptoms are caused by a slow outwards diffusion of small quantities of residual monomer. The upper denture reline must be replaced by one that has been adequately cured to ensure minimal levels of residual monomer.

104 The dimensional changes associated with converting the monomer to polymer using a heating cycle result in the final denture being slightly smaller than the cast. This tendency can be minimised by using the lowest possible curing temperature. The initiation of the conversion of the monomer to polymer by the benzoyl peroxide will take place at about 70°C; any heating above this temperature will have an adverse effect on the dimensional accuracy of the denture base since thermal contraction must occur on cooling to room temperature. High levels of residual monomer can have a deleterious effect on denture base polymers but can be reduced to a minimum by a terminal boil of at least 1 hour.

This terminal boil, however, must not be carried out until the bulk of the monomer is converted or porosity may result. Thus, some compromise is required to obtain good dimensional accuracy, minimal levels of monomer and porous-free dentures. A curing cycle of 7 hours at 70°C, plus 1 hour at 100°C is considered to be the best practical curing cycle. It provides porosity-free dentures, gives residual monomer levels of less than 1.0%, and the additional shrinkage that results from the terminal boil is too small (less than 0.2%) to have any clinical relevance. It should, however, be noted that when using most commercially available water baths it takes more than 1 hour for the temperature to rise from 70°C to 100°C, depending upon the volume of water and the number of flasks being processed. Thus, when using water baths the timing clocks should be set at 7 hours at 70°C (delayed) and 3 hours at 100°C. This curing cycle is satisfactory for all heat-curing polymers and soft lining materials.

See also **11**.

105 (a) The wax-impression technique is used to provide a compressive impression of the underlying mucosa for a distal extension prosthesis. The technique provides stability by preventing the denture sinking and also reduces damaging torque on the abutment tooth.
(b) (i) 'Stress-breaking' designs – split disjunct denture or hinged saddles.
(ii) Precision or semi-precision attachments in the abutment teeth.
(iii) Reducing the size of the occlusal table and fully extending mucosal support of the saddle.

See also **182**.

106 The precentric record is taken when new dentures are being inserted. The purpose is to correct either clinical or laboratory errors that may have resulted in premature occlusal contacts. A double layer of softened modelling wax or silicone occlusal registration material is placed on the lower molar and premolar teeth. The patient is instructed to close in the most retruded position until the maxillary teeth indent the wax or silicone but to stop *before* the teeth contact. Occlusal correction by spot grinding may then be carried out after the dentures have been mounted on an articulator.

See also **29, 110** and **174**.

107 (a) The clinical success of resin-bonded retainers is regarded by many to be inferior to that of conventional full-crown retainers. The most obvious mode of failure would therefore be debonding of the canine retainer. However, this casting is a minor retainer being stress-broken distally by the dovetail connector.
(b) The design would prevent easy maintenance if the canine retainer were to debond. Should this occur then the attachment would prevent easy removal of the mesial retainer. The distal crown and pontic could be preserved as a 2-unit cantilever bridge after cutting the attachment but this would prevent the same design being rebuilt. Alternatively, the whole bridge could be remade.

See also **127**.

108 (a) The lesion is a torus palatinus and, by nature, a benign bony exostosis.

(b) Yes. In this case where the torus is unusually large the denture base cannot cover it and, therefore, the retention is jeopardised because the post-dam is not in its correct position and cannot create the necessary seal.

(c) If the patient is suitable for surgery, then the torus should be surgically removed as part of the treatment plan prior to the construction of a conventionally designed denture.

109 (a) This is a facebow, which acts as a calliper to record the relation of the maxilla to the hinge axis of rotation of the mandible. It enables a similar relation to be established between a maxillary cast and the hinge axis of the articulator. By means of this record, the vertical dimension of occlusion may be altered without repeating the registration of jaw relation.

(b) In prosthetic work, artificial tooth contacts achieved during excursive jaw movements may not be reproduced in the mouth. Similarly, attrition facets and individual tooth contacts present on natural teeth in the mouth may not be reproduced on the articulator.

(c) The simple or arbitrary facebow locates the axis of rotation of an individual condyle head, while a hinge axis or kinematic facebow is attached to a moving mandible and provides recordings of temporomandibular joint movement.

110 (a) The premature contact and lack of coincidence between the retruded and intercuspal positions will cause cuspal interference in function and instability of the dentures. The strain applied to the TMJ by the derangement in occlusion can account for the joint symptoms.

(b) Perform a precentric check record in the retruded contact position and, on an articulator, adjust the recorded occlusion into a new intercuspal position.

See also **29, 55, 106** and **174**.

111 It is essential that the information given to the dental technician is as accurate as possible. Although addition cured silicone materials are extremely accurate, if transfer impression copings are not splinted together there is a risk that there will be some rotational movement and therefore some displacement when the guide pin is released and subsequently retightened onto the analogue.

Splinting of impression copings with a stout metal rod retained by auto-polymerizing acrylic resin or by the use of plaster of Paris reduces the risk of displacement vertically, horizontally or rotationally.

112 This type of denture is called a transitional denture. Teeth may be added to the partial denture as the natural ones are progressively extracted over an extended period of time. This allows the patient to adapt gradually to the wearing of a denture and avoids the shock to the patient of having to adapt to a new denture after the sudden extraction of many teeth.

113 (a) An intraoral Gothic arch or needle-point tracing is being produced, the apex of which indicates the retruded jaw relation of the mandible. The final registration of jaw position is made using impression plaster between the blocks while the point is held at the apex of the tracing.
(b) This method of jaw registration has the advantage of reproducibility in that the position of the obtained apex can be tested as many times as is necessary to confirm its correctness before dismissing the patient. The shape of the tracing reveals the range of movement possessed by the temporo-mandibular joints, with the existence of restrictions and accommodations clearly delineated. Except for contact of the stylus and plate, the occlusal rims do not touch during registration, so occlusal prematurities from this cause are avoided. The stylus and plate assembly also act as a central bearing device, so rims are stable during the tracing and joining together with plaster.
See also **204**.

114 A careful history and examination should have been taken prior to commencement of treatment and, at this stage, some systemic factors may have been identified. If this is not the case, ensure that the lower posterior teeth are not constraining tongue space and that no roughened areas are present on the dentures. Factors such as allergy or residual monomer in the denture base may require investigation, but they are unlikely here as more generalised intraoral discomfort associated with denture-tissue contact would be reported.
If no denture cause is apparent, the patient should be referred to an oral physician, who may perform haematological investigations for iron-deficiency anaemia, folate and vitamin B_{12} deficiencies, and so on. If these are negative, burning mouth syndrome may be diagnosed by exclusion; this has been treated with some success by tricyclic antidepressants.

115 The gingivally approaching clasp on the right premolar is too near the gingivae – trauma is possible in addition to obvious plaque accumulation.

With the anterior saddle, the retention elements for the acrylic are occupying the position of the teeth, thereby preventing a satisfactory match to be made with the natural teeth. It is advisable in such cases to request a wax try-in prior to framework construction so that the technician can see where the denture teeth will be placed, and hence how to wax-up the framework.

116 Although careless handling or injudicious polishing on a lathe may be responsible, the most common cause is occlusal imbalance in retruded contact position. This may be accompanied by a poor fit of the denture base to the palatal tissues. Rebase and re-registration (or a replacement denture) should avoid the vicious cycle of repeated fractures.

117 (a) At this stage the matrices are being located to the patrices and cured into the permanent base *in situ*. This is a clinical or direct location, as distinct from a laboratory or indirect location.
(b) The soft metal spacers are cut and placed over the patrix to cover the root coping exactly, the matrix is then located in position and cured onto the acrylic permanent base using autopolymerising resin. This renders the overdenture tissue-borne, thus reducing the load on the abutment tooth. The clinician then has an added advantage in that the permanent base is positively retained when carrying out the jaw registration at the next visit after the wax rim has been added to the base.
(c) It can be seen that the patient has a congenital cleft palate and, therefore, positive retention using precision attachments is indicated.

118 (a) Investment materials consist of two major components: a binder and a refractory. The two most commonly used investment materials are gypsum-bonded investments and phosphate-bonded investments, which, as their names imply, contain different binders. For a gypsum-bonded investment, the binder consists of an autoclaved calcium hemihydrate, while for a phosphate-bonded investment the binder is ammonium phosphate. Both use a silica refractory.

Gypsum-bonded investments are used for low-melting-temperature gold alloys, and phosphate-bonded investments are used with high-melting-temperature alloys such as porcelain-bonding gold alloys, cobalt–chromium alloys and nickel–chromium alloys.
(b) When a metal casting solidifies and cools, it contracts considerably. The mould needs to be able to compensate for this contraction, otherwise the resulting casting would be too small. This is done by heating the mould to a temperature in the region of 700°C. The material used must be able to withstand these temperatures and, at the same time, expand sufficiently to

compensate for the cooling contraction of the alloy. Both crystobalite and quartz fit these requirements. Fused silica has the thermal stability but shows insufficient expansion on heating to compensate for the contraction of the alloy.

See also **129** and **146**.

119 A distal extension hinged chrome-cobalt connector is illustrated. The hinge is designed to relieve stress that develops on the distal extension from being transferred to the rigid connector on the abutment tooth. The hinge is designed only to allow vertical displacement towards the mucosa while resisting lateral and vertical movement away from the ridge. The initial success of such devices is good but wear on the hinge results in increasing lateral and reciprocal vertical movement, causing discomfort to the patient. A common sequel to wear is the eventual fracture of the hinge.

120 The factors to be considered are:
● The overall physical assessment of the patient and an estimate of the biting force he/she is likely to apply. The greater the load likely to be applied, the shorter the cantilever.
● The prosthetic state of the upper arch. If the lower is opposed by a good natural dentition, substantial, well-supported bridgework or implant-supported bridgework, then the cantilevers should be kept to less than 12mm in the first year to 18 months.
● The arch form of the fixtures. Where fixtures form a flat arch, the anterior/posterior distance between the most anterior fixture and the most distal is of significance. The less this distance, the shorter the cantilever should be. Where the arch is Norman or even Gothic in form, the cantilever can be extended to 12mm or more.

121 The cobalt-chromium maxillary plate has been etched away by solvents. Prolonged exposure to sodium chloride and lactic acid can cause this to happen. It should be noted that the acrylic resin has not been affected by the solvents that have attacked the cobalt chromium. Some denture cleaners contain acids that may corrode metal bases, so patients should be warned of this possibility and instructed never to use household or industrial cleaners.

See also **60** and **198**.

122 A metal-reinforced palate is often utilised in a situation where there is repeated fracture of a conventional upper denture base. Sometimes, repeated fracture indicates poor design or faulty occlusion, and is seen more frequently when there is a full complement of natural lower teeth in opposition. New denture base materials – in particular high-impact acrylics – have been developed, which seem to have overcome some of the limitations of conventional resins, but even so there remain a small number of individuals for whom a metal-reinforced palate is indicated.

While both designs are acceptable, the design of **122A** is preferable since it is easier to develop a satisfactory posterior seal in acrylic rather than in metal. Furthermore, it gives the opportunity for modification at the chairside, particularly where it is the operator's preference to place a physiological seal by means of the addition of autopolymerizing acrylic resin rather than cutting a posterior seal on the master cast, as would be the usual custom. A further advantage is that adjustment is facilitated, particularly where the posterior edge of the denture causes trauma.

See also **172**.

123 A non-precious-metal casting is bonded to the abutment tooth using an autopolymerizing composite luting resin which adheres to the previously acid-etched enamel surface. The components consist of a lingual wing with a rest seat cut in the centre and a proximal extension passing buccally in the form of a small arm. The casting was constructed and bonded to provide support and undercut for a lower removable partial denture. The rest provides support and the proximal arm creates the undercut for a buccally approaching clasp or I-bar. A more aesthetic result can be achieved by using composite resin to provide the same features, but, in time, some wear may lead to a consequent loosening of the denture.

See also **143**.

124 The lower denture has been made on a cast produced from an openmouth impression technique, during which the condyle is displaced forwards and the masseter muscle displaced relatively backwards. During mastication the condyle is in its retruded position, the masseter is in a more forward position and now interferes with the denture base. The notch in the denture base marks the site where the masseter muscle impinges on the lower denture-bearing area.

125 If there is adequate space in the access hole above the screw, a small pledget of cotton wool followed by a gutta-percha plug should be placed before a composite or acrylic restorative material is placed to obturate the opening. If the depth of the hole restricts the amount of material that can be placed above the head of the screw, a small amount of gutta-percha should be placed below the restorative material.

If the access hole is very shallow it may be possible for the patient to keep the space clean without any obturation being attempted. It is important to ensure that no part of the opposing dentition occludes with the screw head.

126 (a) Since the symptoms are related to wearing of the dentures they are unlikely to be caused by a systemic or psychological cause. If the dentures had been inadequately cured, the diffusion out of the residual monomer could give rise to symptoms of this nature. However, observation of the pictures shows that there are small areas of inflammation associated with the lower denture-bearing area and signs that the periphery of the upper denture is traumatising the soft tissues. The most likely cause of the burning sensation is therefore an error in the jaw relations – most probably a lack of freeway space.
(b) The dentures must be replaced.

See also **59** and **103**.

127 (a) Occlusal loads on the canine are directed buccally through the retainer. Buccal displacement of the canine results in bending of the retainer along its length. Resultant tensile stress is therefore concentrated at the proximal ends of the canine retainer, thus causing the resin to fail at this point. Repeated loading extends the point of failure towards the middle of the retainer until it eventually debonds completely.
(b) Tensile loading of resin-bonded retainers should be minimised by using cantilever or stress-broken designs where possible. In this case, a fixed retainer on the second premolar supporting a pontic, linked through a movable connector on the canine, would be best combined with a separate distal cantilever bridge to replace the upper lateral incisor.
(c) The connector on the central incisor was found to be secure. The bridge was sectioned distal to the anterior pontic, thereby allowing the 3-unit posterior segment to be removed. A new stress-broken design was fitted as described above (b) using a resin-bonded, etched-metal–ceramic retainer in the second premolar.

See **107**.

128 (a) A metal-based denture in the patient's oesophagus may be seen on the radiograph.
(b) Small prosthetic appliances may be inhaled or ingested, whereupon they need to be removed surgically. Although the metal-based denture is radiopaque, many prosthetic materials are radiolucent and can be difficult to locate by radiography. Attempts have been made to develop a radio-opaque poly(methylmethacrylate) denture-base resin by inclusion of heavy-metal salts, but no suitable material is currently available.

129 After casting into a mould, the molten metal cools and contracts. Its first contraction occurs between its maximum superheated temperature and its liquidus temperature, during which time there is simply a reduction in height of the still-molten alloy.

Cooling from the liquidus to the solidus states involves solidification and contraction, a process that needs to draw further molten metal from a sufficiently larger, and therefore later solidifying, sprue or reservoir. By means of this provision contraction porosity is avoided.

As it cools from the solidus temperature to room/mouth temperature, the now-solidified casting will again contract. Only the expansion of the investment mould is available to compensate for this contraction. If this is insufficient or is in excess, a dimensionally inaccurate casting will result despite earlier compensations.

See also **118** and **146**.

130 Copy dentures (or duplicate or template dentures) are either provided as replacements for satisfactory dentures, or they are prescribed for patients who have worn dentures satisfactorily for a prolonged period and who will be unlikely to adapt to replacement dentures of a different form. Classically, template dentures may be made for an older patient who has diminished capacity to adapt to dentures with a new form of polished surface.

The existing dentures are replicated by making a template using, ideally, silicone-rubber putty; disposable impression trays may be used to record the polished surfaces of each denture before the impression surface of the denture is replicated. When the denture is removed and returned to the patient, wax is poured into the imprint of the dental arches and self-cure resin is poured via ingates into the mould to copy or replicate the polished surfaces. After the removal of blemishes, an accurate impression of the denture tissues may be taken with silicone rubber. At the same visit, the occlusal tables may be modified by the addition of wax. Before the next clinical visit, acrylic teeth are set up in the positions indicated and satisfactory form and function are determined prior to finishing.

131 (a) The 3 mechanisms involved in creating a bond between the metal coping and the porcelain are:
(i) Mechanical retention.
(ii) Compression.
(iii) Chemical bonding.

Mechanical retention takes place as the porcelain flows into the microspaces in the surface of the metal. On cooling, the metal will try to contract more than the porcelain by virtue of its higher coefficient of expansion. In doing so it leaves the porcelain in a state of compression which is highly beneficial for this brittle material. A chemical bond is created between the porcelain and the oxide coating on the metal. During firing, the molten glass fuses with the oxides on the metal surface as the oxides migrate into the porcelain.

(b) It is important that the mismatch in the coefficients of thermal expansion is small, otherwise the internal stresses created during cooling could cause the porcelain to fracture. The most likely place for such a failure is at the interface between the metal and the porcelain.

132 (a) This is because if a buccal flange was present and extended normally, it would have to be constructed on a blocked-out working cast to make insertion possible. The flange would then create a large food trap and cause an unsightly bulge above the abutment teeth.
(b) The missing flange weakens the denture structure and is often the cause of fracture of the base in the region of the abutments.
(c) If the overdenture has to be designed so that the flange over the abutments is omitted, then it is wise to consider a cast cobalt–chromium base to provide the necessary rigidity.

133 (a) Denture granuloma or denture-induced hyperplasia.
(b) Chronic pressure from an old, ill-fitting denture or from an overextended denture will cause hyperplasia of the soft tissues. If an ulcer forms, the infection that follows will cause additional swelling as a result of the associated inflammation.
(c) Relief of the denture in the affected area will remove the source of chronic trauma. Any associated ulcer will then heal and the inflammation will resolve, with consequent reduction in size of the mass. If near-complete resolution occurs so that the remaining mass does not interfere with function, new dentures can be made. When a substantial mass of unresolved fibrous tissue remains, it must be removed surgically.
See also **12**, **86** and **192**.

134 Simple hinge articulators, which allow only an opening and closing movement, unfortunately are still widely used. By only considering the occlusion in retruded closure and excluding protrusive, retrusive and lateral excursions, dentures constructed in simple-hinge articulators will be unstable in any excursion away from retruded contact position. It is not possible for the technician to 'grind in' the teeth to accommodate these excursions, so extensive intraoral occlusal adjustment would be necessary by the dentist to correct the problem.

The use of fixed condylar-angle articulators allows protrusive, lateral and possibly retrusive excursions to be made. The teeth can also be placed, adjusted and ground in to allow these excursions to be made. The fixed condylar angle can cause a problem, and is usually set at 30° on each side. Dentures made on these articulators cannot possibly be identical to, or match the patient's own condylar angles. Therefore, slight instability can be expected and some intraoral occlusal adjustment may be necessary. When using an articulator with adjustable condylar angles, it may, in certain instances, be possible to record the patient's own condylar path angles using a mandibular facebow, or by the use of protrusive and/or lateral check bites, and to transfer these angles to the articulator. Dentures made on such articulators would then reproduce the patient's own movements more accurately.

Simple-hinge articulators cannot be used with a facebow. Fixed and adjustable condyle-angle articulators can be used with a facebow, allowing the casts to be mounted on the articulator in the same relationship to the articulator condyle heads as they are in the patient.

See also **32**.

135 When using average condylar angles (30°), Christensen's phenomenon (a parting of the posterior teeth in protrusive movements) may occur, leading to tipping of the dentures. By placing a lower right premolar on the left side (and vice versa) behind the last molar, it allows the upper last molar to contact it during protrusive excursions, therefore maintaining balance. This tooth should be placed slightly higher than the occlusion and will need to be 'ground in' by the technician/dentist.

See also **158**.

136 It is essential for the surgeon to appreciate the intended size, position and angulation of the artificial teeth. The prosthodontist must indicate to the surgeon where and at what angle fixtures should be placed when using the stent, a device that is easily applied during surgery. It is sometimes better to avoid placing a fixture rather than place one where it would intrude on an interdental space.

A stent indicating the position of the teeth and, in particular, the incisal edges, requires good access to the palatal tissue for the surgery, as shown in the illustration. An alternative would be to use a silicone putty mould of the labial aspect of the anterior teeth, extending it round to the premolars to provide stability.

If possible, the prosthodontist should be present at the time of surgery to allow the surgeon to consult on matters that may not be evident until the time of operation.

137 (a) Alveolar resorption over the last 15 years has reduced the occlusal face height. This, in association with wear of the incisor teeth and loss of restraining overbite, has produced the condition of protrusive overclosure. (b) Before attempting to increase the face height to an acceptable value, it is necessary to evaluate the extent to which a person of this age can adapt to the change in jaw relations. Small additions of self-cure resin to the occlusal surfaces of the lower posterior teeth can be used to produce gradual increases in face height without going beyond the patient's limits of adaptation. When a tolerable increase has been produced, new dentures can be made to the increased face height. A form of denture duplication may be used to ensure that changes in the shape of the polished surfaces and tooth position do not cause the dentures to be rejected.

138 A steep incisogingivial curve has been produced on the pontic, thereby creating shadowing at the cervical margin. This results from an attempt to match the length of the pontic with that of the neighbouring incisor. The choice of shade is reasonably good but is spoilt by poor contouring. The incisal edge of the pontic is slightly short and has been rounded at each end. The proximal contours taper steeply and do not match the adjacent incisor outline. Metal is visible in the mid-line. The proximal and incisal edge errors are easily corrected by careful refabrication of the porcelain. The poor buccal contour is more difficult to correct and will depend on the height of the smile line of the patient.

If the smile line is below the gingival margins of the upper teeth then the labial contour of the pontic could match the adjacent natural incisor to make the pontic much longer than it is at present but the increased length would not be visible. If the smile line is high, then the possibility of soft-tissue recontouring or ridge augmentation should be considered as the loss of soft tissue is significant in this case.

139 Clinical and/or technical faults are often responsible for patient dissatisfaction with dentures. Anatomical factors frequently make it difficult to provide satisfactory dentures, e.g. gross alveolar resorption and strong musculature often cause problems. However, psychological problems and unrealistic expectations may also be factors.

The plastic bags containing dentures and spectacles suggest a particularly poor adaptive capacity. The prognosis for satisfactory dentures is poor. New dentures that are technically correct may be provided but a particularly sympathetic approach is needed, along with an explanation of the difficulties of adaptation and the limitations of function. Referral for specialist advice may be necessary.

140 Although internal resorption cannot be excluded, the discoloration is most likely organic in nature and a result of pulp-degradation products entering dentinal tubules. In the case of organic discolouration, internal bleaching is very successful but a prerequisite is a well-condensed root filling. Once the root canal has been obturated, the coronal access cavity is enlarged in order to remove any residual pulp tissue and pulp-horn remnants. The internal dentine surface should be etched to open up the dentinal tubules. The etching also facilitates bleaching with 30% (100vol) hydrogen peroxide under the rubber dam, this being placed in the pulp chamber on pledgets of cotton wool and activated by either heat or light. The process is repeated a number of times and the tooth sealed with a pledget of cotton wool moistened in hydrogen peroxide. The process may have to be repeated on a number of occasions.

Since bleached teeth sometimes discolour further with age, re-treatment may be necessary. It is therefore important not to obturate the whole pulp chamber by means of a composite filling material but instead to use dentine-coloured gutta-percha internally as this facilitates potential re-treatment. Following this, a conventional composite restoration can be placed to seal the coronal access cavity.

See also **34**.

141 Success of a denture constructed in such a situation depends upon good support, retention and stability. Hypernasal speech and fluid leaks can be embarrassing. In this instance, as the defect is acquired rather than congenital, these potential drawbacks may be overcome with careful technique.

The denture would generally be fabricated so that a bulb engages the defect (from which some retention might be obtained). Whether the denture is constructed in 1 part or 2 with a separate 'bung', taking an impression of such a defect can often be difficult.

A useful technique is to take an incremental impression of the defect using silicone putty. The first stage is to adapt a portion of putty to the mesial and distal aspects of the defect. When set, these are removed, liberally coated with petroleum jelly and re-inserted. Putty is then applied to the medial lateral aspects of the defect and, once set, these too are removed, coated in petroleum jelly and reinserted, and a final increment of putty is then added. The number of increments needed varies. Once set, an overall impression is taken over the putty-filled defect to include the residual ridge.

Upon removal, the putty 'jigsaw' is cleaned and reassembled using a cyano-acrylate cement. This is located on the overall impression, which, if taken in a custom tray, forms the working model. Once poured and after all impression material has been removed, the master-cast accurately depicts the residual ridges and their relationship to the defect, whose internal anatomy will also be reproduced accurately. The working cast may then be used to fabricate a 1- or 2-piece obturator and, if necessary, the defect can be adjusted by blocking out so that the appropriate amount of undercut is engaged, taking care to avoid sensitive vital structures such as the nasal turbinates.

See also **97**.

142 In the edentulous jaw, the correctly installed implant has some latitude of required position. For the single tooth in the front of the mouth this tolerance is virtually non-existent. The greatest possible accuracy of implant position and angulation is necessary. Severe, if not impossible, technical problems are caused by the misplaced single-tooth implant with, at best, emergence angle and crown length both severely compromised. Because the necessary prosthetic components are of an unalterable size, the space available in the mouth for these must be measured accurately. When this space is at a premium, even slight lateral implant malpositioning means that a crown cannot be made in the space provided.

143 There are no undercuts on the teeth anterior to the saddles and these will need to be modified – for example, by the addition of composite or resin-bonded metal undercuts. Rest-seat preparations are necessary and the casts should be articulated to determine space available for the clasp assemblies and so on. The opposing teeth may also need to be modified.
See also **123**.

144 This is an immediate-insertion denture with an open-faced design. Socketing has been incorporated in this denture and, unless this is removed, scalloping of the residual ridges may result. To reline this denture, any undercuts should be removed, the open face should be eliminated by the addition of greenstick compound or wax and, following confirmation of the post dam and peripheral seal, a reline impression should be taken using an appropriate material such as zinc oxide – eugenol. Should the labial undercut be excessive or the patient reject a flange and accept a reduction in retention, then a ridge-lap design should be used and the greenstick moulded to the convexity of the ridge prior to the reline impression.

145 (a) The implant is placed in 2 separate surgical procedures. Part 1, called the fixture, is placed so that it is in intimate contact with a threaded hole drilled in bone. When correctly installed, the fixture is entirely contained within the outer cortical plate of the bone. This is the fixture onto which new bone is formed to produce what is known as osseointegration.
After healing and confirmed osseointegration, an abutment (part 2) is screw-connected to the fixture at a second operation. The gold cylinder (part 3) forms the interface by which prostheses are connected to the implant. When cylinders are included in prostheses they form a fixed restoration; when attached to implants external to the prosthesis they form the basis of a retention system for an overdenture.
(b) External threads are necessary to provide fixture stability immediately after their installation and during the earliest stages of osseointegration.

(c) Precious-metal frameworks are more predictably cast on to gold cylinders. Casting on to titanium is unreliably difficult for present casting technology.

146 Control of pre-casting mould cooling. Moulds must be removed from the furnace and placed in a casting machine so they will cool from their design temperature before casting. This cooling occurs at a faster rate and is accompanied by a greater contraction than that occurring during furnace heating. As a result of this heat loss, the interval of pre-casting mould cooling must be kept to a minimum by pre-heating (but not melting) the metal prior to mould removal from the furnace. The shorter the pre-casting mould cooling interval, the greater the fitting accuracy of castings.

See also **118** and **129**.

147 (i) Construct the prosthesis and obturate the access cavities with a composite restorative material.
(ii) Change the abutments to angled abutments on 1 or all of the fixtures.
(iii) Construct a cast-gold alloy subframe with machined lateral surfaces to receive a close-fitting casting retained by secondary screws, clips or a locking device, and onto which prosthetic teeth are processed.

148 Such patients often complain that the upper denture is loose, particularly in function. Frequently, they give a history of having been provided with a partial lower denture but of having been unable to wear it. Thus, loading anteriorly on the complete upper denture causes tipping and displacement, breaking the posterior seal. Frequently, the soft tissues underlying the anterior portion of the upper denture are somewhat displaceable; this is thought to be a result of increased loading causing trauma, this in turn leading to excessive resorption of the residual ridge.

Examination of the patient's existing dentures, including the lower partial denture (even if not worn), is often helpful. In most cases, inability to wear a partial lower denture indicates poor design and can often be overcome. Treatment must aim to provide well-designed dentures; this requires careful technique and consideration of occlusion and occlusal relationships. Patient education is also required on the need for a lower partial denture.

See also **49** and **94**.

149 (a) Die coatings are used with the intention of providing a space between the casting and the prepared tooth that is sufficient to accept an adequate thickness of cement lute. For this reason, coatings should not extend onto the fitting margins/shoulders of preparations.

Since the recommended maximum thickness of luting cement is only 25µm, the use of these coatings implies great accuracy. With this cement film thickness in mind, the applied coatings should presumably be at or less than 25µm in thickness. Damaged coatings and damaged dies beneath these coatings, especially when accompanied by ground fitting surfaces of castings, are important findings.

(b) The die illustrated indicates that internal fitting errors may exist which are sufficient to prevent complete seating of the casting, and/or that the cement lute will have an increased thickness.

See also **57** and **191**.

150 (a) Retention can be defined as the resistance to forces that tend to displace the denture in an occlusal direction. Stability is the resistance to movement in a horizontal direction.

(b) The factors that determine the retention of complete dentures in the mouth are essentially physical in nature. Anatomical factors such as undercuts may be a nuisance rather than an advantage since the denture is rigid and cannot engage hard undercuts. In some instances this might require pre-prosthetic surgery to remove the undercut.

Adhesion of the denture to the mucosa is provided by the saliva, and the greater the surface area, the better the adhesive bond. At the same time, it is important that the cohesion of the saliva film is not destroyed; this is best guarded against by having as thin a film of saliva between the mucosa and denture as is possible. Very important to the retention of the denture is the establishment of a peripheral seal around the edge of the denture. As patients get older, the rate of production and the consistency of their saliva may change so that it becomes less adhesive to the denture and less viscous. It is particularly important to consider the use of drugs that reduce salivary flow.

151 (i) Twin-mix technique. In this technique the wash is mixed and syringed around those prepared teeth for which an accurate impression is required. The putty is mixed and placed in the stock tray. The loaded tray is then inserted in the patient's mouth and the 2 impression materials allowed to set together. Upon removal, there will be some deformation of the impression material, most of which is recovered immediately by a recoil action. If the cast is poured virtually immediately, little or no shrinkage from storage contraction of the impression material will have taken place, and the resultant cast will be only slightly bigger than the tooth as a consequent of polymerisation shrinkage and cooling contraction. If the pouring of the cast is delayed, then, depending on the length of time of the delay, the resultant cast will be bigger in the case of the condensation-cured silicone because of contraction on storage. As the addition-cured silicones are extremely stable on storage, the cast will be of the same size no matter when it is poured.

(ii) Two-stage with spacer technique. Effectively, this technique involves the production of a special tray with the putty being used first. A primary impression is taken either directly on the oral surfaces or sometimes with a thin cellophane sheet laid over the putty. In the case of the former situation, the poor-quality impression of the teeth is cut out, thereby creating a channel for the wash material. A second impression is then produced using the wash, this providing the necessary surface detail. Generally, more of the wash material is required in this technique than with the twin-mix approach, and this means that there is more polymerisation shrinkage as the wash has a much lower filler content. This is especially true with condensation-cured silicones, these also showing more shrinkage on storage. The addition-cured silicones are relatively unaffected by such problems. Also, with addition-cured silicones the need to remove a stiff putty material from undercuts is avoided using this method.

(iii) Two-stage without spacer technique. In this technique the first impression is taken with the putty. The wash is then placed around the teeth and in the tray containing the set putty, and reseated in the mouth. This process of reseating can itself by quite problematical. As a certain amount of space is required by the wash there will be some compression of the putty to accommodate this. The excellent recovery of the silicone-impression materials means that immediately the material has set and is removed from the mouth, there will be a recoil action as the pressure on the putty is relieved. If a cast is poured virtually immediately, the recoil action of both impression materials is likely to be slightly smaller than that of the tooth. For the condensation-cured silicones, the shrinkage on storage will ensure that after a delay of 24 hours this situation will have reversed. However, the addition-cured silicones are so dimensionally stable that the cast will always be too small.

152 (i) The space between the roots of the adjacent teeth must be adequate enough to ensure that placement of a fixture will cause no damage to the root surfaces or periodontal membranes.

(ii) There must be adequate clearance for instrumentation during the placement of the fixture. This clearance is normally 7mm.

(iii) There is adequate bone present so that a fixture can be placed deeply enough to permit the correct emergence angles for the crown.

(iv) As removal of adjacent tooth tissue will be necessary, full assessment of the resultant aesthetics must be carried out with trial wax-ups.

153 (a) The enlarged maxillary tuberosities prevent adequate posterior extension of the upper denture, hence adequate posterior peripheral seal. The tuberosities also occupy the space that might otherwise be occupied by a lower partial denture, which itself would provide support to the upper denture and prevent the lower anterior teeth acting to destabilise the upper denture.
(b) Surgical reduction of the maxillary tuberosities.
  See also **46**.

154 (a) Angular cheilitis.
(b) Yes. It is usually associated directly with denture-induced stomatitis. This inflammatory condition is normally localised to the denture-bearing mucosa of the complete upper denture. The denture is ill-fitting, the hygiene is poor and the appliance is often worn 24 hours a day. Bacteriological investigation may reveal the presence of *Candida albicans*.
(c) The patient should be advised to limit denture wearing to essential times only during the day and improve the standard of oral hygiene. It is advisable to prescribe an antifungal agent and apply a tissue conditioner to the denture base to improve the fit and also to help resolve the inflammation in the underlying mucosa. When the problem has resolved, a new complete denture will be designed which should help to restore both the fit and the support of the lips and the corners of the mouth to acceptable contours.
  See also **6**, **59** and **194**.

155 Calculus build-up around the fixtures, which has spread along the prosthesis. It may be avoided by:
(i) Thorough oral-hygiene instruction and maintenance.
(ii) Regular scaling by the dentist/hygienist using plastic-only instruments.

156 Careful questioning in a situation such as this is important, since without a proper diagnosis treatment may fail. Tooth-surface loss is often associated with dietary factors – for example, excessive intake of fruits, particularly of the citrus variety. One must be aware that acids can be 'hidden' in the diet – for example, acetic acid and lemon juice. Acetic acid is often used in association with French fries and pickles. Other sources of extrinsic acid are carbonated drinks, of which some cola varieties are notorious because of their phosphoric acid content. However, other carbonated drinks should not be ignored, particularly when it is noticed that they are taken regularly and to excess. The peculiar habit of cleaning teeth with lemon juice should also be considered as a possible factor.

Having excluded extrinsic sources of acid, one must look elsewhere. Gastric reflux, possibly associated with a hiatus hernia, chronic alcoholism or bulimia are all possible factors.

Where the cause of the tooth-surface loss is extrinsic, careful dietary advice is often all that is required, particularly when patients realise the damage that they are causing to their teeth. Where there is gastric reflux, the advice of a medical practitioner should usually be sought, particularly in cases of bulimia where special counselling may be required.

Assuming there has been no compensatory over-eruption of opposing teeth, the treatment of choice might be restoration by means of dentine-bonded porcelain laminate onlays. Alternatively, conventional crown restorations may be indicated and, depending upon the extent of loss of tooth substance, elective devitalisation may be required prior to placement of post crowns.

See also **161** and **183**.

157 In principle, an article is formed from a molten glass by the lost-wax casting process and a metastable glass results on cooling. During subsequent heat treatment, controlled crystallisation occurs with the nucleation and growth of internal crystals. This conversion process from a glass to a partially crystalline glass is called 'ceramming'. Thus, a glass-ceramic is a multiphase solid containing a residual glass phase with a finely dispersed crystalline phase. The controlled crystallisation of the glass results in the formation of tiny crystals that are evenly distributed throughout the glass.

158 (a) Called Christensen's phenomenon, this wedge-shaped space is caused by the condyle heads descending their respective glenoid fossae. Since the space is a product of condylar inclination, this effect may be made use of to form a protrusive record wafer. This can then be used to adjust an articulator's condylar guides with registrations of the patient's individual condylar inclinations.

(b) A space between the posterior teeth is avoided in complete dentures by arranging these teeth in a curve related to left and right condylar guidance, cusp angles of the teeth, incisal guidance and the plane of orientation. Called the compensating curve, it is analogous to a combination of the curves of Spee and Monson.

See also **135**.

159 A silicone-putty index may be made from the master-cast, placed palatally and grooved by a guide-pin, reduced in length to 2 threads and placed in the hole for the gold screw. This guide-pin may then be used to support the abutment firmly in place while tightening the abutment screw.

160 (a) The abutment teeth remained vital because of the slow process of tooth wear. The teeth were then simply domed and smoothed using diamond instruments, with about 1mm of sound tooth supragingivally. Care must be taken to eliminate any undercuts about the gingival margins.
(b) Not in this case, since the overdenture has complete palatal coverage and, therefore, conventional means of retention are quite adequate even though the overdenture had to be designed without a full labial flange.
(c) The labial flange was contraindicated for 2 reasons:
(i) The labial undercut was too deep.
(ii) The labial undercut would have distorted the lip unnecessarily.
  See also **22, 85, 95, 165, 169** and **188**.

161 We must assume that the periodontal and gingival conditions are satisfactory prior to restoration of the dentition. Since there may be a parafunctional element and treatment might involve an increase in occlusal vertical dimension, the wearing of an occlusal splint (constructed at an increased occlusal vertical dimension) would be a suitable starting point. Alternatively, a conventional upper partial denture overlaying upper molars and onlaying 321|123 with tooth-coloured and contoured resins might be a better choice, and will also allow satisfactory aesthetics and occlusion to be developed. This should be in combination with a lower partial denture constructed to the existing lower occlusal plane. Ultimately, assuming satisfactory progress with the partial denture, the anterior onlay can be cut away as upper anterior teeth are crowned to the new occlusal vertical dimension. Finally, upper molar teeth may be crowned and a conventional, toothborne partial denture constructed to fill residual tooth spaces.
  See also **156** and **183**.

162 A custom tray with wire loops is used to enable a neutral zone impression to be taken.
  The neutral zone or zone of minimal conflict between tongue and cheeks is recorded in order that the stability of the lower denture may be optimised. The technique enables the position of the polished surface of the denture to be defined and the artificial teeth to be placed in an area of minimal muscular activity.
  See also **17**.

163 If the vertical dimension was correct at the time of the try-in, then this error will have occurred during 1 or more of the denture-processing stages as follows:
• Trial dentures were incorrectly returned to their casts before investing.
• Inaccurately fitting flask parts.

- Weak investing plaster was used, allowing mould distortion or tooth movement during flask closure.
- Resin packed in too hard a consistency, thus forcing teeth into the investing plaster.
- Air pockets are present in the plaster into which teeth can move.
- Flask halves not sufficiently pressed together, thereby allowing a resin membrane or flash to increase denture thickness.

164 Tilted implants have no advantages. Depending on their severity, tilted implants can provide almost insuperable difficulties for prosthetic care. In this instance, it is certain that screw access holes will appear within the labial or buccal surfaces of the teeth. These can usually be satisfactorily obturated at the chairside by the use of tooth-coloured filling materials.

More difficult is when access holes insist on protruding through incisal edges, this producing aesthetically unacceptable notches in the teeth. Severe technical difficulties arise when the implants form angles greater than about 35° with each other. The prosthesis–implant connection interface will then not allow prostheses to be installed in the mouth. Angulated abutments may be substituted but even these will not correct implants as severely tilted as shown. Individually made gold cylinder and/or abutment parts, the use of only those implants capable of realignment by angulated abutments and the construction of prostheses in pieces are difficult last-resort options in these cases.

165 (i) The upper right canine has been root-filled and restored with a post and root-face coping. The occlusal surface of the coping has been flattened to contact a magnetic attachment fitted in the prosthesis.
(ii) A high-coercivity permanent magnet is encased in a thin titanium housing that is retained in the prosthesis. When fully seated, the magnet rests on the cemented casting, this being made from a 60% palladium, ferromagnetic alloy. The strong 'open field' magnet is retained against the cast-alloy keeper until a load in excess of 300g is applied. A single path of insertion has been provided by the other abutment restorations, therby ensuring displacement only with vertical forces.

See also **22, 85, 95, 160, 169** and **188**.

166 (i) It must spread the forces acting on it evenly over the supporting tissues. This should be within their physiological limits and the denture should be adequately retained in position in the mouth during all functional movement.
(ii) It must prevent the dental arch from collapsing by preventing the teeth from drifting or tilting into edentulous spaces. It should cause minimum damage to both soft and hard tissues.

(iii) It must maintain the health of previously unopposed teeth by restoring them to function and preventing their over-eruption.

(iv) It must restore masticatory efficiency and appearance, and also be comfortable to wear.

(v) It should restore or maintain occlusal vertical dimension, and prevent dysfunction of the temporomandibular joints.

167 This is the most universally quoted classification system. Kennedy does not classify the completed denture but the unrestored condition of the mouth. There are 4 classifications, the first 3 of which may show 1 or more modifications.

- Class I. Tooth loss is bilateral and extends posteriorly to the remaining teeth. This classification is one requiring treatment by a denture having 2 free-end saddles. A modification would be added to the classification if a further bounded saddle were present; such a case would be referred to as Class I modification I.
- Class II. Tooth loss is unilateral and again lies posterior to the remaining teeth. This classification is one requiring treatment by a denture having 1 free-end saddle. Modifications may also be added as with Class I.
- Class III. Tooth loss is unilateral with teeth anterior and posterior to it (a bounded saddle). Treatment is by a denture with a unilateral bounded saddle. Modifications can also be added.
- Class IV. Tooth loss is entirely anterior to the remaining teeth. Treatment is by a denture with only an anterior-bounded saddle. This classification has no modifications, the reason being that if there were a modification it would revert to one of the other classifications, the anterior saddle becoming a modification.

168 The upper teeth have obviously been placed on the residual ridge and provide little in the way of lip support. In consequence, a disproportionate amount of tooth is shown. Little thought has been given to independence of tooth form and gingival contour is conspicuous by its absence. More posteriorly, an obvious step is seen between canines and first premolars; no buccal corridors are visible. As a consequence of poor placement of the anterior teeth, inverse posterior occlusal curves are present. In addition to compromising appearance, the latter will also compromise function.

169 These teeth have been altered to serve as overdenture abutments. They have undergone elective endodontics, which avoids bulky cores that restrict tooth height and denture aesthetics, as well as adding bulk to the prosthesis. In addition, where teeth have not been reduced, acrylic-based overdentures are prone to fracture. Should additional retention be required, it is relatively easy to prepare stud or bar precision attachments to teeth prepared in this way.

See also **22, 85, 95, 160, 165** and **188**.

170 Dental implants are unattractive in appearance and do nothing to aid speech or mastication; this is not their function. Implants are foundations for future prosthetic care and it is only the promise of an enduring and stable prosthesis or restoration of minimal bulk that justifies the use of implants.

171 The spaces between the denture periphery and the palatal aspects of the natural teeth can only lead to food packing and its sequelae.

172 (a) To create a stronger than normal base where there exists a history of fracture of previous acrylic-based dentures caused by heavy occlusion.
(b) This is a cobalt–chromium alloy base which is ideal to resist fracture because of its rigidity. Careful scrutiny of the base will show the observer the detailed fitting surface that is typical of a casting.
(c) Swaged stainless steel is occasionally used for complete upper denture bases where problems of tolerance, because of the thicker acrylic base, have caused problems. The thin stainless-steel base is well tolerated and is a good thermal conductor, thereby creating a more natural and desirable effect for the patient.
(d) Metallic-based dentures cannot be relined and rebased easily.

See also **122**.

173 (a) The patient has a repaired bilateral cleft lip and palate; the premaxillary segment of bone is underdeveloped.
(b) Precision attachments have been chosen to give the prosthesis positive retention because conventional retention would be unsightly and also ineffective in preventing anterior displacement. The precision attachments provide the major proportion of the anterior retention and can be augmented by conventional clasping on the posterior teeth.
(c) Other forms of restoration would be contraindicated because of the gross anterior alveolar loss. The overdenture allows the clinician the freedom to set the anterior teeth in a favourable position in relation to the lower teeth and the upper lip in a situation where the occlusion is usually abnormal.

174 (a) The problem is almost certainly occlusal in origin, probably a premature contact in the anterior region. When the dentures are brought into occlusion firmly, the upper denture tips down at the back by means of a leverage effect.

(b) The dentures may be mounted on an articulator by means of a pre-contact check record and the occlusal surfaces adjusted.

See also **29**, **55**, **106** and **110**.

175 (a) (i) Contraction porosity. This porosity occurs since the monomer will contract some 20% by volume during processing. By using the powder/liquid system, this contraction is minimised and should be in the region of 5–8%. However, this appears not to be translated into a high linear shrinkage, which on the basis of the volumetric shrinkage should be of the order of 1.5–2% but is in fact somewhere in the region of 0.2–0.5%. It is believed that this is because the observed contraction is primarily caused by thermal contraction from the curing temperature to room temperature and not the curing contraction. At the curing temperature the resin remains sufficiently fluid to contract at the same rate as the mould, this being aided by the pressure that is exerted. The resin only becomes rigid once it gets below its glass transition temperature, at which point the curing contraction will have been completed. From this point on it is the thermal contraction that contributes to the observed changes in dimensions of the denture base.
(ii) Gaseous porosity. On polymerization, there is an exothermic reaction that could cause the temperature of the resin to rise above its boiling temperature – just above 100°C. If this temperature is exceeded before the polymerisation process is completed, gaseous monomer will be formed. The amount of heat generated will depend on the volume of resin present, the proportion of monomer and the rapidity with which the external heat reaches the resin. The formation of gaseous porosity can be avoided by allowing the temperature to be raised in a slow and controlled fashion.

It is important that sufficient dough is packed in the mould such that the material is under pressure while being processed. This will cause any voids present in the mix to collapse and also help compensate for the curing contraction. Thus, the packing of the mould should only be carried out when the mix has reached the dough stage.
(b) Polymerisation must be carried out *slowly* (to prevent gaseous porosity) and *under pressure* (to avoid contraction porosity).

See also **11** and **48**.

176 Prosthesis–implant connecting screws should be sufficiently tightened so that they are stretched just short of their yield point. By this degree of tensioning, screws are removed from further loads up to the value of the applied pre-load, are protected and their service life is extended. An accurately calibrated torque wrench is essential for this work.

In the absence of this tool, some implant manufacturers design screw-driver handles so that a maximum amount of finger-tightening obtains an acceptable screw pre-load.

See also **83**.

177 Many such patients exhibit classically worn occlusal planes and have resultant postural protrusion with accompanying decrease in occlusal vertical dimension. The acquired protrusive posture may be habitual and retruded contract position (RCP) may be difficult to obtain. While conventional methods of intermaxillary registration may yield reproducible results, in problem patients occlusal pivots have been used with some success. The lower denture has 2 pillars of autopolymerising acrylic that are placed on the pivotal area (second premolar, mesial half of the first molar) of the lower denture. These pillars serve as a 'bite-freeing' splint and enable the patient to adopt a muscularly determined RCP.

In intractable cases, replacement dentures may be provided in the form of pivots until a reproducible RCP is recorded.

178 A partially edentulous mouth has many undercuts. An undercut can be defined as an area that is out of contact with any vertical dropped from a given horizontal. Denture bases and rigid parts of clasps will not pass into undercuts. It is therefore important for the designer of a partial denture to be able to identify these areas.

179 (a) Calcium sulphate hemihydrate – dental plaster, gypsum plasters.
(b) (i) High-fusing porcelain.
  (ii) Low-fusing porcelain.
(c) Gold-casting alloys:
  (i) Soft.
  (ii) Medium.
  (iii) Hard.
  (iv) Extra hard.
(d) (i) Sticky wax.
  (ii) Modelling wax.
  (iii) Inlay wax.
(e) Alginate impression material.

180 (a) The posterior teeth on both sides of the denture have been placed lingually to the centre of the ridges. The teeth are therefore unsupported and, as masticatory forces are exerted, mid-line fracture could occur. Before this outcome is reached, lower denture instability may have been experienced due to tongue 'cramping', soreness of the mouth and a loss of occlusal balance during function.

(b) It is essential for the stability of mandibular dentures on poor ridges to place the teeth over the centres of the ridges so that maximum support and stability are obtained. The positioning of the upper teeth in such cases can be slightly compromised to ensure correct mandibular tooth placement.

See **69**.

181 Good oral hygiene is obviously desirable for any prosthesis and the age of the patient may influence the type of restoration. Patients younger than 16–18 years are generally not considered for conventional bridgework and it may be considered unwise to place a fixed restoration in a young adult who is actively engaged in contact sports such as karate or rugby. The number of missing teeth may also influence the type of restoration, or may preclude any restoration! Spacing may indicate pre-prosthetic orthodontics prior to restoration with fixed or removable prosthodontics. Measurement of bone quality and quantity may indicate that an implant may be considered, although, as with all restorative options, occlusal factors must be assessed.

See **184**.

182 (a) It has always been a problem to produce accurate working casts for mandibular distal extension removable partial dentures. Ideally, such casts should record the edentulous areas and the remaining teeth in functional relationships similar to those that will occur during occlusal loading.

A 2-tray system enables functional displacement of the denture-bearing tissues to be obtained. An impression technique that causes such displacement of the tissues will enable a removable partial denture to be constructed that will reduce leverage on the abutment teeth and provide even pressure on the edentulous areas along their entire length.

The primary impression is made in a close-fitting acrylic resin tray with zinc oxide/eugenol paste, the functional denture-bearing tissues being recorded. The remaining teeth and tissue areas are then recorded using a spaced acrylic-resin special tray with a polysiloxane-type impression material. This latter tray also covers the handles of the first tray so that similar functional pressure can be exerted on the first impression as the second is made, the 2 trays being locked together by the second impression and removed from the mouth as one. The working cast produced from such an impression technique will reproduce all tooth surfaces and the denture-bearing tissues in the functional state in which they would be positioned when the removable partial denture is in place during mastication.

(b) The most commonly used method of creating a functional relationship between teeth and tissues in mandibular distal extension, removable partial dentures, is the altered cast or 'Applegate' technique.

This method allows a corrective impression to be made of the functional denture-bearing areas in a small personalised tray made around the retentive elements of the metal partial-denture framework. This can be made in either zinc oxide/eugenol paste, impression wax or polysiloxane impression materials. The old saddle areas of the cast are then cut away, the denture base and new impression are relocated on to the cast and the new impression is poured with dental stone and allowed to attach itself to the old cast.

See also **105**.

183 This is a moderately early case of tooth surface loss. The enamel, particularly labially, is somewhat featureless and this suggests that there may be an element of erosion. Tooth wear may also be associated with a parafunctional habit and careful assessment is required in order to identify possible aetiological factors. Where the source of acid is diet-related, careful counselling and advice is often all that is required. Where there is gastric reflux, the advice of a medical practitioner should be sought, particularly in bulimia where special counselling may be required.

Where aesthetics are basically satisfactory, treatment should aim at preventing further damage. Topical fluoride and fluoride mouthrinses help, strengthening the enamel surface and making it more resistent to acid attack. Where there is a parafunctional habit, there may be a need to provide a nocturnal splint.

At this early stage, advice is often all that is required but, in order to identify further deterioration, clinical photographs and study casts are very helpful. These provide a baseline from which to make a future comparison in order to identify ongoing change. Regular review is therefore important and requires a well-motivated patient. With early intervention as described above, more drastic forms of treatment involving protracted and costly restorative care can often be avoided. Early diagnosis and counselling is important if future problems are to be avoided.

See also **156** and **161**.

184 The upper arch, which is shown in isolation, is moderately heavily restored. Assuming that the occlusion is favourable and that potential abutment teeth are minimally restored, one option would be the placement of an adhesive bridge. Rather than construct this as a fixed–fixed bridge, evidence suggests that a cantilever restoration may be more successful in the long term.

Given that the canine is heavily restored, it is not an ideal abutment for an adhesive bridge and conventional bridgework would be the treatment of choice. The lateral pontic might be cantilevered off the canine but this would first require a full assessment. Factors to be considered include the shape of the clinical crown and crown length, periodontal support and occlusion in lateral and protrusive excursions. Apart from providing a 'centric stop', care should be taken to ensure that the pontic is not loaded in other excursions. Loss of labial bone and the associated soft-tissue defect labially in the lateral incisor region is likely to compromise aesthetics by making it difficult to achieve a satisfactory relationship of pontic to soft tissue. In such circumstances, it may be possible to augment the defect with a synthetic-bone substitute such as hydroxyapatite prior to provision of the bridge.

See **181**.

185 (a) This problem is seen most commonly in the lower jaw where there is a smaller surface area over which to distribute the load and where patients may have a sharp, thin or heavily resorbed alveolar ridge. If the pain persists when all measures have been taken to minimise the occlusal load, the denture may be made more comfortable by the use of a soft liner. This provides a means of absorbing some of the energy involved in mastication by interposing a highly resilient material between the denture and the mucosa, thus spreading the load more evenly over the soft tissues.

(b) Two major types of soft lining materials are silicone rubber and acrylic-based materials:

(i) Silicone-rubber soft liners. The silicone-rubber soft liner consists of a polydimethyl siloxane polymer, to which is added a certain amount of filler to give it the correct consistency. The material solidifies by a cross-linking process. This can be achieved both with heat (using benzoyl peroxide) or chemically (using tetraethyl silicate).

(ii) Acrylic soft liners. Polyethyl methacrylate is the main constituent of many soft liners. It has a glass transition temperature (Tg) of only 66°C, compared with 100°C for polymethylmethacrylate (PMMA). A combination of this polymer with a small amount of plasticiser (such as dibutylphthalate) is enough to bring down the Tg sufficiently to produce a soft material at mouth temperature.

(c) Silicone-rubber soft liners do not bond readily to the acrylic resin of a denture and an adhesive needs to be employed. This can consist of a silicone polymer dissolved in a solvent or an alkyl-silane coupling agent. In either case, the bond is very weak and usually fails within a relatively short time. Also, this material tends to support the growth of *Candida albicans*, which may lead to denture-induced stomatitis. This limits the life of such bonds to 3–6 months.

The acrylic-based soft liners have the advantage that they bond well to a PMMA denture. Unfortunately, the plasticiser gradually leaches out and the liner becomes stiff as it loses its resilience. The speed at which this transition takes place depends to some extent on the patient's regime for cleaning the denture. In general, high temperatures should be avoided.

186 The cast surveyor consists of a flat horizontal platform, attached to which is a rigid vertical column with a movable hinged arm suspended from its top. Dropped from this arm is a vertical rod which can be moved up or down and locked in any position. The end of this vertical rod is designed to hold instruments. Also attached to the main horizontal table is a multi-movement table with some form of clamp to hold the cast rigidly. The tools used with the surveyor are:

● The analysing rod. This is used for the preliminary examination of the cast and to determine the correct path of insertion.
● The carbon marker. This is used to mark the most bulbous part of the tooth and tissue undercuts when the correct path of insertion has been found.
● The undercut gauges. These are 0.01, 0.02 and 0.03 in or 0.25, 0.50 and 0.75mm gauges. They are used to measure the amount of undercut present and accurately locate the position of the depth of undercut required for any given clasp.
● The wax and plaster trimmer. This is for removing excess wax and plaster that has been used to block out unwanted undercuts.

These tools are held in the instrument holder of the vertical rod. The instruments are held in a vertical position and can be moved over the cast using the swinging hinged horizontal arm. The cast attached to the movable model table can then be tilted at any angle to the vertical instruments.

See also **3, 79, 193** and **200**.

187 The lower anterior teeth are positioned too far anteriorly to the residual alveolar ridge to be in the neutral zone. In function, the denture will be displaced by the pressure of the labial musculature in this region. Passive opening of the mouth will have the same effect.

188 The advantages of overdenture therapy are:
(i) Firm support is provided for the denture by the exposed root surfaces.
(ii) Less alveolar resorption occurs and greater stability results from the greater amount of alveolar bone – fewer relines may also be required.
(iii) There are psychological benefits to the patient, who feels that all is not yet lost.

(iv) It has been claimed that adaptation to the dentures may be quicker and easier if the proprioceptive reflexes in the periodontal membrane are preserved.

The disadvantages are that:

(i) Root canal therapy may sometimes be difficult due to the variable root canal anatomy.

(ii) The bone mass surrounding the root buccally may produce an undercut that will compromise appearance.

(iii) Caries and periodontal disease can occur in the stagnation area beneath the overdenture. It is essential to emphasise good oral- and denture-hygiene habits. Topical fluoride should be applied regularly at home and fluoride varnishes applied at recall visits in the surgery.

(iv) Since more alveolar bone is retained, the overdenture is usually thinner than a conventional complete denture. Fracture is therefore more common and permanent overdentures may often include cast-metal bases for increased strength.

See also **22, 85, 95, 160, 165** and **169**.

189 (a) Fracture in ceramics is usually initiated from a small surface or internal defect such as a micro-crack, this acting as a stress raiser. With the inclusion of a crystalline phase in a glass, the size of these micro-cracks can be limited to the region between the crystalline particles. Thus, the smaller the crystals and the larger the volume fraction of the crystals, the smaller the cracks will be and consequently the greater the strength of the material.

(b) A number of additional strengthening mechanisms are open to exploration with ceramics. These strengthening mechanisms rely on the formation of a compression layer on the surface and include the following:

(i) Ion-exchange. The surface of the material can be placed under compression by replacing some of the metal ions with larger ions via an ion-exchange mechanism. The compression of the surface layer is achieved by the changed volume of the exchanged ions.

(ii) Heat treatment. A compressive surface layer can be formed during cooling by blowing cold air on the surface of the ceramic. This causes the outside layer to contract more rapidly than the interior. When the outside layer has cooled to room temperature, the interior continues to try to contract, thereby placing the surface under compression.

(iii) Surface glass. If a surface glaze with a lower thermal expansion than the bulk ceramic is fired on to its surface, a thin layer along the surface will be under compression once the material has cooled.

190 (a) The amount of spacer used when constructing special trays is directly related to the type of impression material that will be used in the tray.

Normal denture wax used to provide a tray spacer has a sheet thickness of 1.5mm.

Impression materials have different physical properties: some can be used in very thin section (zinc oxide paste); while others would be too weak in thin section (alginate) and would not recover accurately when removed from undercuts. The latter therefore need to be in thicker section.

For alginate impression materials, 2 layers of spacer to give a 3mm thickness are used. Impression plaster requires 3 layers of spacer wax 4.5mm thick in total to enable accurate relocation of any broken pieces of impression on removal from the mouth.

Elastomeric impression materials require 1–2 layers of spacer 1.5–3mm thick, depending on whether a light- or heavy-bodied material is to be used. Zinc oxide pastes are required in very thin section as they are used to record edentulous mouths with no severe undercuts. They therefore require no spacer wax, the special tray being made directly on to the cast.

(b) The materials available for the construction of special trays are:
- Self-curing acrylic resin.
- Heat-curing acrylic resin.
- Shellac-base plate.
- Light-curing materials.

Self-curing acrylic resin is widely used, strong, fairly cheap, easy and quick to manipulate, it is also easily adjusted in the mouth. It is suitable for use with all types of impression materials.

Heat-curing acrylic resin is not widely used, is time-consuming to make and is more expensive but it has similar properties to self-curing acrylic resin.

Shellac-base plate material is widely used, is weak, is easily distorted in the mouth, is brittle and will easily fracture. It is not suitable for all impression materials but is cheap and fairly easy to manipulate.

Light-cured materials are relatively new. They are easy to manipulate with minimum finishing required, they are strong, easy to adjust in the mouth, are probably the quickest material from which to make a tray and can be used with any impression material. However, they require an expensive light-curing unit for polymerization.

(c) Alginate impression materials need to be mechanically locked to the impression tray; adhesives will not work efficiently on their own. To provide mechanical retention, holes are drilled into the tray starting 3–4mm from the periphery of the tray, then 2mm-diameter holes are drilled every 10mm around the tray in ever-decreasing circles 10mm apart.

The excess alginate material will squeeze through the holes during the impression-taking and, after setting, will lock the impression material to the tray.

See also **23**.

191 (a) The first fault seen is called 'cold lapping'. This is where the wax pattern has not formed a solid coating against the die, one layer of molten wax not having blended with another, and thereby leaving a split between them. This fault is most commonly seen towards the shoulder of a restoration.

The second fault is a number of 'cast nodules' attached to the fitting surface of the casting. These are caused when air is trapped between the wax pattern and investment during the investing process, the air bubbles subsequently filling with molten alloy.

(b) Cold lapping causes a lack of fit and can also cause a weakness in the casting, usually at the crown margins. This weakness, combined with a possible slight distortion of the metalwork during the porcelain application, can lead to a loss of marginal accuracy.

The cast nodules would prevent complete seating of the crown and could cause damage to the core of the tooth. Up to 50% of cast nodules inside castings cannot be seen by eye alone, magnification being required. Careful examination and removal of such nodules should be carried out by both the technician and dentist before fitting.

See also **57** and **149**.

192 This is denture-induced hyperplasia. It is fibrous tissue associated with trauma caused by an overextended base. The trauma is usually a result of alveolar resorption which causes the denture to settle onto the tissues. An unbalanced occlusion may cause an unstable denture base to tip and traumatise the mucosa.

The denture periphery should be cut away from the hyperplastic tissue. The denture should be left out as much as possible. If resolution is not sufficient, residual tissue should be excised. If a considerable amount of tissue is to be excised and extensive sulcus loss is anticipated, a limited sulcoplasty should be considered. Excised tissue should be sent for histological examination. Ill-fitting dentures should be replaced following resolution or surgical excision.

See also **12, 86** and **133**.

193 (i) To locate the height of contour lines on teeth for a given path of insertion.

(ii) To determine the best path of appliance insertion and removal for each individual partial denture.

(iii) To measure the amount of undercut present on a tooth and therefore the actual position of a clasp arm, taking into account resiliency of the metal to prevent trauma to the teeth or breakage of the clasp.

(iv) To determine soft tissue and tooth undercuts that must be blocked out prior to cast duplication or denture production.

(v) To identify soft-tissue undercuts that may require surgical removal or be used for added retention when compatible with the path of insertion.
(vi) To provide information for the design of the entire partial denture, including clasp design and position, the location of occlusal rests and the location of bars and plates.
(vii) To aid in determining the restorative procedures necessary on abutment teeth.
(viii) To trim wax patterns of crowned teeth to coincide with the path of insertion, improve the fit of the appliance and aid reciprocal action.

See also **3, 79, 186** and **200**.

194 This is a denture-induced stomatitis and is related to the fitting surface of a partial denture. Although the usual cause is a combination of trauma from a denture, it may occasionally be due to an allergy to the denture base. Treatment should include:
(i) Reduction of trauma to the mucosa.
(ii) Leaving dentures out at night.
(iii) Oral hygiene of mucosa and dentures.
(iv) Antifungal treatment.

See also **6, 59** and **154**

195 This is a training plate and is recommended for patients with a history of retching. The need to ensure a good peripheral seal and intimate contact with palatal tissues is paramount, although no occlusally derived instability should be present. It may be necessary to provide a double post-dam in case the patient cannot tolerate an adequately extended post-dam overlying the palatine aponeurosis.

196 (a) When relining such a denture at the chairside, it is essential that the following precautions are taken:
(i) Block out the matrix so that the mechanism is not rendered inactive by the reline material flowing around it.
(ii) Ensure that the matrix is fully seated on the patrix during the recording of the reline impression. This will ensure that the matrix still fits precisely on to the patrix following the relining procedure.
(iii) Ensure that the denture is in the correct occlusion during the relining procedure.
(b) Depending on the alveolar resorption rate, the overdenture inevitably becomes toothborne on the abutments. If this goes unnoticed, the increased load causes the following:
(i) Overloading of the periodontal tissues of the abutments.
(ii) Stresses in and around the matrices in the denture, resulting in their

possible dislodgement, fracture of the attachment matrix or fracture of the denture through the abutment zone. Any overdenture is inherently weak in the abutment area because of the space occupied by the matrix, and also by the reduced bulk of the denture base as a result of the abutment tooth and alveolar bone surrounding it.

197 This patient has received hydroxyapatite augmentation of the mandibular ridge, presumably as denture-wearing was difficult. In addition to problems associated with any surgical procedure, problems may be both short term and long term. Short-term problems include possible infection, tenderness, avoidance of denture-wearing for approximately 4 weeks and possible paraesthesia. Long-term problems include migration of granules, loss of granules and mucosal dehiscence.

198 Patients should be made aware of the plaque-retentive potential of any prostheses, and thus regular removal and cleansing of these dentures and the patient's mouth are of paramount importance. As the prosthesis shown has a cast cobalt–chromium base, it should not be soaked in hypochlorite or other such reducing solution as the passifying oxide layer may be imperilled. The patient should be instructed not to place the dentures in boiling water as, in addition to possible warpage of the denture, the acrylic may be bleached.
See also **60** and **121**.

199 Possible causes here are subdivisible into the following broad categories:
(i) Related to supporting tissues. Check for retained roots, unerupted teeth, cysts and so on. Radiographs should be taken. Also check for ulcerated areas that may or may not be denture associated and palpate for any knuckles of bone, knife-edge ridges or displaceable tissues. Such palpation helps identify any areas of atrophic mucosa overlying healthy bone. In addition, check for a superficial and palpable mental nerve.
(ii) Related to the denture base. Palpate the base to detect sharp ridges of acrylic or pearls of acrylic. Ensure that the denture-supporting tissues are adequately covered by the denture base – underextension increases the pressure on the area covered! In cases where support problems are present, have appropriate impression techniques been employed? Check for overextension of the denture periphery. Although strictly speaking this is not a support problem, the resultant instability may result in discomfort.
(iii) Related to occlusion. Occlusal imbalance may result in pressure and/or instability and should be corrected. It is essential that bilateral even contacts exist in retruded contact position (RCP) in all patients receiving replacement complete dentures.

200 (a) (i) Kennedy Class I. With bilateral free-end saddles, premolar abutment teeth often have undercuts on their distal surfaces (next to the saddles). In situations like this, the cast could be tilted anteriorly to eliminate the undercuts. Any denture made to this path of insertion would in effect fit into this undercut and help to resist vertical dislodging forces placed upon it during function.

(ii) Kennedy Class IV. In this case we have an anterior saddle. It would be usual to tilt the cast posteriorly to reduce undercuts on the mesial aspects of the abutment teeth. This has the effect of eliminating unsightly gaps between the denture base and teeth in order to improve aesthetics.

In both the above cases, all the unwanted undercuts must be blocked out with the cast in these positions on the model surveyor.

(b) Undercuts fall into 2 categories:

(i) Wanted undercuts. These are those that may be used to provide retention for the partial denture.

(ii) Unwanted undercuts. These are those that interfere with the fitting of partial dentures.

Having found the most suitable path of insertion and designed the denture, the unwanted undercuts should be blocked out (filled with either plaster or wax). This is done using the plaster and wax trimmer on the surveyor. Plaster is used for permanent work and wax for temporary work. The plaster or wax is placed into the undercut and the trimmer used to remove excess material, so the undercut is neither under- nor overfilled.

(c) When the clinician has designed a partial denture, he needs to be able to transfer the cast to the technician. The clinician must show the technician the exact tilt or orientation on his surveyor to enable the technician to achieve the same position on his surveyor. This can be achieved by placing the analysing rod into the surveyor and then placing it against the side of the cast base. A pencil is used to draw a line down the analysing rod on to the cast, this being done at the back of the cast and down each side.

On receipt of the cast, the technician will place it on the surveyor table and adjust it until the lines down the base correspond to the analysing rod in the surveyor. The cast table can then be locked into this position and the subsequent work can then be carried out with the path of insertion chosen by the dentist.

See also **3**, **79**, **186** and **193**.

201 This is a heat-cured silicone-rubber resilient lining. It is added to freshly cured acrylic and is not recommended in patients with candidal infections or xerostomia. If the mental foramina are superficial, the technician should be instructed to relieve these areas of the cast, otherwise a plug of silicone rubber may flow into the foramen with resultant neuropraxia.

See also **185**.

202 The radiographs demonstrate hypercementosis, and the bulbous nature of the roots would suggest difficulty with extractions. This appearance, along with the pulp canal calcification, is suggestive of tooth wear (and attrition in particular).

203 The further the flanges of a partial denture saddle extend into the functional sulcus, the greater the stability and resistance to horizontal displacing forces at right angles to the flanges. With a lower partial denture, maximum extension of the flanges should be a requirement with anterior saddles and free-end saddles because of the small surface area available for support. In the upper jaw there is greater flexibility due to the support available from the palate. With an anterior saddle, variations may depend on the number of teeth being replaced, the cosmetic result, the shape of the palate and the degree of undercut of the labial sulcus.

204 This is the arrow-point tracing or Gothic-arch tracing technique. It can clearly be seen where the retruded contact position (RCP) is found, it is reproducible and it is made by the patient without manipulation by the clinician. In addition, pressure is equalized on the supporting tissue in both jaws owing to the fact that the only contact between the mandible and maxilla is a centre-bearing point on the opposing plate.
   See also **113**.

205 It is possible to obtain a graphical recording of condylar inclination so that direct measurements can be made for setting the condylar elements on the articulator. Restriction in movement and lateral deviation during protrusion may be seen, and differences in condylar inclination between the 2 sides can readily be identified.

206 (i) In order to direct forces down the long axes of the abutment teeth.
(ii) To ensure a satisfactory fit of the rest on the tooth that is less noticeable to the tongue.
(iii) To enable the polished surface of the rest to have a shape in harmony with the anatomy of the tooth and the functional occlusion.

207 The speed with which the tooth wear has taken place. With slow wear over a number of years, the pulp chambers and canals decrease in size in response to the aetiological factors. Rapid wear does not allow time for this to occur and such teeth become sensitive.

208 (i) Fixed bridgework.
(ii) Removable partial denture.
(iii) Attachment denture.
(iv) Implants.

209 A denture can restore the contour of the arch labially and provide satisfactory lip support more effectively. In addition, in situations like this the teeth may have been lost due to trauma, with concomitant loss of alveolar bone. Under normal circumstances bridgework cannot replace bone, and hence cosmetics may be compromised.

210 In **210A**, the patient is closing in retruded contact position (RCP). In **210B**, the mandible has postured forwards and the patient has overclosed in order to get a functional contact of the posterior teeth.

211 Some form of parafunctional habit, such as biting of hairgrips, nails, pen tops and the like.

212 This is the split-cast technique. It is a method by which a cast can be removed from the articulator and then replaced in exactly the same position. For example, processed dentures can be remounted after deflasking and the occlusion refined to take account of processing errors before removal from the cast. When examining the occlusion, if casts are mounted in retruded contact position (RCP), the upper one can be removed and placed in intercuspal relationship (ICP) with the lower in order to see the discrepancy between the 2 positions.
See also **11**.

213 The incisor relationship and the fact that the lower anterior teeth contact the upper ridge mean that great difficulty would be experienced when providing a removable partial denture, a fixed bridge or implants.

214 The patient has obviously been wearing the dentures for many years without any maintenance. The lower denture has sunk into the lower ridge, the clasps traumatising the gingival tissues. The patient has then started to posture forwards to gain a posterior 'functional' occlusion and has ended up with a Class III incisor relationship.

215 Apart from the poor cast preparation generally, part of the denture-bearing area has been fractured and then badly repaired. The denture is unlikely to fit satisfactorily.

Index

Numbers refer to question and answer numbers.